UNF*CK YOUR MIND

Shatter Your Limiting Beliefs to Become Who You Were Meant to Be

JANNA JOHNSON

LANDON HAIL PRESS

Copyright© 2024 Janna Johnson
All Rights Reserved

This book or any portion thereof may not be reproduced or used in any manner without the express written permission of the publisher, except for the use of brief quotations in a book review.

Paperback ISBN: 978-1-959955-26-9
Hardback ISBN: 978-1-959955-27-6
Cover design by Rich Johnson, Spectacle Photo
Published by Landon Hail Press

Although the author and publisher have made every effort to ensure the accuracy and completeness of information contained in this book, we assume no responsibility for errors, inaccuracies, omissions, or any inconsistency herein. Any slights on people, places, or organizations are unintentional. The material in this book is provided for educational purposes only. No responsibility for loss occasioned to any person or corporate body acting or refraining to act as a result of reading material in this book can be accepted by the author or publisher.

I dedicate this book to every single experience that created the limited mindset, beliefs, and wounds that I once had but that were necessary to happen for me to become the person I was meant to be. I wholeheartedly dedicate this book, this labor of love to Brady, Bryndle, and Broden, my 3 precious kids. One day you will be old enough to read this book. May this book be a teacher to you that you cannot give anyone or anything your control. Allow adversity to be your teacher and never live in the past. Every experience you have is meant to shape you but only if you allow it. Lastly, thank you to all of those close to me for your constant support, love, and encouragement.

CONTENTS

FOREWORD _____ 1
PROLOGUE _____ 4
INTRODUCTION _____ 9
CHAPTER 1: Who the Fuck Am I to Write This Book? _____ 13
    This Book Was Supposed to Be About… _____ 20
CHAPTER 2: Break Out of the Safety Box _____ 25
    Judging Others is Your Defense Mechanism _____ 32
CHAPTER 3: The Birth of My Limiting Beliefs _____ 35
    Growing Up _____ 40
CHAPTER 4: The Fire of Sadness Blew Up in Flames _____ 47
    False Confidence _____ 51
    Naïve and Deceived _____ 54
    Fresh Start, Same Wounds _____ 58
CHAPTER 5: The First Catalyst of Breaking the Chains _____ 64
    Rock Bottom _____ 71
    Pure Determination _____ 74
    Time to Die _____ 76
CHAPTER 6: The Cost of the Victim Mindset _____ 83
CHAPTER 7: Perfectionism is a Mask _____ 90
    My Body Became My Garbage Can _____ 97

- CHAPTER 8: The Eye-Opening Final Catalyst — 102
  - Fuck This Shit — 105
- CHAPTER 9: Surrendering: The Beginning of Change — 112
- Chapter 10: Create the Space — 121
  - Pull the Weeds Out! — 124
  - Get Rid of Unneeded Pressure — 126
  - Boundaries — 129
- CHAPTER 11: Rejection — 133
  - Time to Listen to a New Tape — 136
  - Desires Meet Action — 139
- CHAPTER 12: Taming Your Inner Beast — 147
  - High Expectations — 154
- Chapter 13: Parenting: With or Without Chains — 158
- CHAPTER 14: Time to Choose — 165
  - Stop Accepting and Start Choosing — 168
  - Stop Attaching Your Happiness — 170
- CHAPTER 15: The Path to Freedom — 175
  - Get Real Uncomfortable — 179
- CHAPTER 16: Say Yes to You! — 187
  - The Power of Alone Time — 193
  - Reflection — 198
  - Choose You — 201
- ACKNOWLEDGMENTS — 207
- ABOUT THE AUTHOR — 209

FOREWORD

IF YOU KNOW ANYTHING about Janna Johnson, it should come as no surprise that my friend has written *UnF*ck Your Mind*. That's because she has been able to shatter her own limiting beliefs, rise from the ashes, and is now an example of experience, strength and hope for others!

The instant I met Janna I knew she was a force for good in the world. The more I got to know her, I knew her message would be life changing, *Especially* for those who need hope and inspiration.

Janna is fearless. She never wavers, and she is relentless in studying what it takes to succeed. By extension, Janna is fully invested in sharing that knowledge with others so they, too, can become who they are meant to be.

None of us knows what our particular brand of struggle will be in this life. We often encounter unexpected challenges, from the shadows of illness to the relentless storms of negativity. It is during these trying times that our resilience is truly tested.

This book is a compass for those navigating the difficult terrain of pain, illness, negativity, feeling stuck, have hit roadblocks or even rock bottom. It is a guide crafted with authentic empathy and wisdom that will take you from having a victim mindset to being the victor of your life.

As you embark on these pages, you'll discover not just strategies for survival, but how to truly thrive. You will learn to shift your mindset, take back your power and have the freedom to go after your big dreams. It provides pathways to true transformation.

Janna shares her own stories of triumph over adversity, lessons extracted from the darkest moments, and the profound strength that arises from confronting the seemingly insurmountable.

This isn't just a collection of words; it's a testament to the resilience of the human spirit. It explores the power of mindset—the often-overlooked force that can shape our realities.

Each chapter is a step forward, an invitation to embrace the potential for growth even in the face of despair.

This book is a source of inspiration, a reservoir of hope, and a roadmap for anyone seeking to emerge stronger and unstoppable.

As you delve into the profound insights within, may you find the strength to rewrite your narrative and emerge from life's tribulations not merely as a survivor but as a beacon of resilience and positivity.

The journey ahead is yours to navigate, and within these pages lie the tools to forge a mindset that transforms challenges into opportunities, darkness into light.

Take your time with Janna's words. Keep a pen in hand. And savor the gracious gift she has given to us in this book.

UNF*CK YOUR MIND

Discover for yourself how you can completely shift your mindset and live the life you have always imagined!

Here's to a journey of healing, growth, and the unwavering strength that lies within us all.

With Love,

Amberly Lago, Bestselling Author of *True Grit and Grace*
Top-Rated Podcast Host of *True Grit and Grace*
Motivational Speaker

PROLOGUE

"You are so stupid and dumb. You will never amount to anything. If it wasn't for me, you would work a minimum-wage job at best. You didn't even graduate college. Look at everything I have given you, and you are so ungrateful! Do you know how many women would give anything to have what you have and be in your shoes? Hell, if it was up to you to earn an income to take care of this family, we would live in a shack. Thank God people actually like me and I know how to make money. Just shut up, sit there, and look pretty. You can do that, right?"

I CAN AND I WILL. It isn't worth me doing anything else, after being put down and demeaned into nothing, I will be lucky if I can muster a smile. Thank you so very much for constantly reminding me how you think of me, all because I am inquisitive and try to understand things.

What is it about me that attracts this behavior? Do I really sound dumb? I wish I wasn't so misunderstood. I do know one thing: you don't talk to people you love that way. I don't have the ability, and I just don't understand.

For my entire life, as long as I can remember, I have never felt good enough, smart enough, or pretty enough. Right here in this very moment, as I sit in the car on the way to an event, I know this is the most painful it has ever felt. God, *why? What is wrong with me?* I am a good person. I am honest, loving, loyal, kind, nurturing, and I can't stand to see anyone hurting. So why, God, do I have to be treated this way? Have I not done enough? Was Lyme disease not enough pain and torture?

When am I ever going to get a fucking break? Because I feel like I will break, if I don't get one! I wipe the tears away before they are noticed. I control my breath before it is apparent that I might be crying. I reach into my purse to check my makeup, like I always do before I get out of the car…

"Fuck!" he barks. "You are not fucking crying, are you? God damn, I can't take you anywhere. You are so embarrassing."

Deep breath, Janna.

"I am not crying. I am simply checking my makeup, like I always do, and I have never embarrassed you, so don't worry about me. All is well."

"You know that you bring this upon yourself, right? I mean, put yourself in my shoes. I bust my ass, working and providing, and all you do is take and complain. If roles were reversed, you would feel the same, but we both know that it is all up to me to be the provider. And I am the only one who can make money. Just be grateful. *Smile* and be *nice*, if you can even do that. I know it's hard."

Thank God we finally pull up, and he is done tearing me to pieces. And there he goes, talking to his friends by the door, still smiling and talking about how good his day was. *Wow.* I feel even smaller now. I just want to go home. I am worn the fuck out with being done this way.

Maybe I *am* fucking stupid and worthless, but I don't think so. I don't want to get out of this car! I just want to go home to cry and scream!

What did I ever do to deserve this? And anyway, I know I am not the person he's choosing to spend time with. Why am I putting up with this? The hopes and dreams I have, deep-down inside, on top of my intuition, all nag at me constantly that I *do have a purpose here on this Earth*!

All I know is that I can't bear this emotional pain and heartbreak for one more second! I am tired of fighting for someone who won't fight for me, for someone who behaves like they want to be with someone else. *Am I really not good enough to fight for?*

Oops, he's actually looking to see if I am out of the car yet. Better put that fake fucking smile on, swallow my sadness, and go do my part. Lord knows it's not for me.

*****

Moments like that happened far too often. Were there also good times? Sure, of course. But I don't care how many "good times" there are. There should *never* be one of the times I described above.

My fear and what my gut had been telling me for eighteen months was indeed really happening. I was pretty sure that my heart was being ripped out of my chest and put in a blender. I was mad at God. This emotional pain was unbearable. I had to leave and get out of the house.

This was the *most* painful time of my life. I couldn't eat, smile, or laugh. I barely drank water. I just sat alone for six days with myself. I cried until I had no more tears left. I relived every single painful, hurtful moment in my life. I felt every bit of it.

My heart was in a million pieces. All of the pain and hurts I had ever experienced came to a head; I could take no more. Maybe I needed to be completely broken.

I decided then that I was *done* being told what to do, what to say, or that I wasn't enough! I wanted to go after my dreams! It scared the shit out of me, but I was ready to say *yes* to *me*! I knew that the road ahead of me, along with the major changes and transitions were going to be tough, but this was the road I'd been put on. I either walked forward into the unknown, absolutely terrified and not having a clue where to start, or I walked backward into the weeds that were growing over me, trying to pull me in. The anger and pain inside of me were the pressure needed to be applied in order to push me into wanting freedom.

Thank goodness I walked forward. You see, a lot of people just keep going backward, looking in the rearview mirror. You cannot get to your true destination that way. I had no clue what was ahead of me on this new path that I had not only been placed on, but then had *chosen* to take. I already knew what was in the rearview mirror. But what was in front of me?

Those six days alone were pivotal for me, because I finally saw the patterns. I clearly saw that the Universe was trying to show me something. *What*? Yes, it sucked what had happened. *No*, I did not deserve it or any of the other brutal times in my life. I couldn't change what happened or who was responsible for them. But I had an awakening that showed me I had been living my life as a victim.

I was constantly reacting, doing, saying, or choosing from a place of limiting beliefs and mindset. For my entire life, I had believed every single lie and criticism. I was the one standing in my own way! I had allowed the wounds and hurts of my past to continue to hurt me and bleed on me every day! No more! It was time to get my power back.

I knew it wasn't going to be easy, but I was ready to find out who I was, to love and accept myself, and to go after everything that scared me. I was and am the only one who can make my dreams come true!

You hold the power to your success. The key to unlocking it is in shattering those limiting beliefs that created a limited mindset, and then you are free!

INTRODUCTION

IT IS QUIET AND YOU ARE ALONE, reflecting and wondering why you're not living the life you desire deep down for yourself? A life so fulfilling, confident, and happy, filled with endless opportunities. If only we could hit a pause button, reassess, revise, and hit play again.

Unfortunately, no such thing exists. Time keeps on ticking by, and in the blink of an eye, another year has gone by. The question is, why is your life stagnant and unfulfilling? Why is nothing changing for you for the better? There are invisible chains each of us have with a limiting belief attached to each one. Those chains are holding you back from living the life you dream of.

I can't thank you enough for picking my book to read. Trust that you are exactly where you need to be at this very moment. Please know that writing this was a labor of love and my gift to you. I poured my heart out, sharing the most painful moments I have ever been through, and being unapologetically authentic in every word you are holding.

The purpose of my vulnerability and honesty is to help others overcome, heal, and step into their purpose here on

Earth. You are not meant to live an unfulfilling, unhappy life of constant struggle.

What drew you to my book? Are done feeling like a hamster on a hamster wheel? Feeling like you are living day after day on autopilot? Let's be honest: what really drew you to this book is curiosity. There is a feeling deep down in the pit of your stomach that quietly nags at you, whispering that you could live the life you want, could fulfill your dreams, have true happiness, and feel free!

So, what is stopping you from listening to your gut? My guess—and this is what I used to think—is you believe your dreams and desires are silly. You are defeating yourself mentally, telling yourself that your dreams are stupid or unachievable, before you even try! You are not giving yourself a chance. No one else will take a chance on you, if you cannot even give that to yourself.

You have become a prisoner in your own mind, to your own thoughts. Frustration about wanting so much more in life consumes you. You are stuck because you are scared. The same old shit and the same types of people seem to always show up, constantly triggering you and keeping you in the rabbit hole, so there is no way your life will ever be any different.

Do you know your triggers? Many of us do, but the real question is why do you have the triggers you have, respond the way you do to certain situations, and make the decisions you make? Your thought processes and mindset are the result of every pivotal moment since you were born. That is exactly what you will learn in this book. What it looks like living with limiting beliefs, unhealed wounds, and trauma, but also what it looks like after you shatter them! You can break free from the invisible chains holding you back and the ghosts from the past that haunt you. I did. It is 100% possible; the power lies in you! When you break free from your limiting beliefs, heal, shift your mindset, and stop living in the past, you can become all that you were meant to be!

I am not just sharing stories from my past while staying at the surface level of the memories. No, I am retelling painful memories, staying true at the very core of reality. My spirit has been tested beyond what I thought possible and broken, only to rise again. On this journey of my own life, you will see how it has been shaped by the birth, consequences, and shattering of limiting beliefs. You will learn the consequences I suffered from living with invisible chains and a limited mindset, as well as the resilience and willpower necessary to shatter those chains and limiting beliefs. In the pages ahead, you will walk with me on my journey through my most dark and painful times, which tested and shattered me into a million pieces, allowing me to put myself back together, but without the pieces that did not serve me well.

We will explore the roads filled with insecurities, self-doubt, fears, and the pressures we allow others and society to put on us, creating roadblocks to our true selves.

I will teach you how I uncovered my limiting beliefs, tracing each one back to its root, and the exact footprint for how I cut the invisible chains and pulled each limiting belief up by its root. I rose from the ashes of the fires trying to burn me, if I let them, or prepare me for my true purpose.

Let this book teach you and prepare you for your own journey ahead of you. Open your mind to all of the possibilities waiting for you with a limitless mindset. Reading my transformation and being able to compare what my life was like with limiting beliefs versus shattered beliefs will empower you to do the same for yourself, so you step into your power and purpose.

Stop ignoring that strong pull, deep down in your core, that there is something you are called to do in your life. You do not even need to know what your purpose is, but you know it is waiting to be uncovered. You are in the right place. You are holding the keys that set me free from the personal prison I had put myself in. This is a guide that teaches you how to set yourself free from the past and pain that are holding you back.

There is nobody else in this *entire* world like *you*! Not one. Sure, there are a lot of similar people, but not the exact same. Two people can share the same environments and experiences, but each one will process it differently and be affected differently. We all have our own unique footprint that makes us special.

Your mindset is the greatest tool you have! It is the *ultimate weapon* and the *deciding factor* for how you will live, for your success, healing, overcoming, love, happiness, and the influence you have on your kids.

We are not meant to just survive through life, but to *thrive*! We worry too much about how not to die, but it is time to give just as much energy to how to *live!* Are you ready to *Unf*ck Your Mind?*

*****

CHAPTER 1

Who the Fuck Am I to Write This Book?

One day, I realized I was waiting on someone else to make my dreams come true. I looked in the mirror and knew I was the only one to make it happen, so I went for it!

WHY SHOULD I WRITE this book? Who the hell am I to think I can or that anything will come of it? So, you went through something dark and painful? Everyone does. It doesn't make you special. You were never good enough growing up, at least so you thought, and you have never felt good enough at forty-one years old, so you had a few moments over these last eight months, when you finally took a chance on yourself, but you're not even fully confident. You are scared. You are not good enough. All the hopes and dreams you have of what you could become, of what you want to become, well, they are just hopes and dreams and always will be...

    That is me, talking to myself. The nagging voice in my head daily, which reminds me of who the hell I am and also keeps me safe. The voice that keeps me from making a fool of myself.

The voice that keeps me down. The voice that, for forty-one fucking years, hasn't done one goddamn thing except to hold me back and make me cry like a baby. The voice I always thought was my voice of reason. Or was it?

Hmm, well, I still listen to that voice. I just did. But now, when I hear those haunting words, I see them as a reminder of everything I will go after and achieve. There are days when that voice makes me procrastinate and wonder if I am even worthy or good enough. But that is a far stretch from what it used to do to me.

That self-defeating voice was a part of my life for way too long. I remember the moment I realized it was just a *voice!* It was not the *truth!* I never realized that that voice was a tape, playing over and over in my head, created from my life experiences, beginning in my childhood; it was the way I interpreted and reacted to them, internally. There were hurtful painful memories that had not been healed.

Until you realize that that nagging voice is not the truth or reality but rather your insecurities and limiting beliefs stemming from painful moments from your past, then you will continue to listen to it and live by it. But that is holding you back from being who you are meant to be and living your purpose.

What voice is playing in your head? If you were to think about anything you have really been wanting to do for yourself, what is the first thing you hear in your mind?

Do you hear, "No, you can't do that!"

"It won't work out!"

"What are you thinking?"

Or, "Everyone will laugh!"

If you hear any of those phrases, then please do not think that is logic or truth! Those are phrases of self-doubt and fear created from your limiting beliefs. That is where that tape was created that constantly plays in your head, just like it did mine. You also probably think that voice is keeping you safe from failure. It is *not* keeping you safe from failure. It is blocking you from growing into your true self!

How are limiting beliefs created? Why is it you tell yourself the things you do?

We are constantly thinking about something. Did you know we have somewhere between 40,000-60,000 thoughts a day? Now get ready for this... Around eighty percent of thoughts are negative! Wow! If that isn't-eye opening enough, how about the fact that most people *accept* the first thought that enters their head! Do you ever stop to wonder if maybe what you are thinking *isn't true?*

Or do you believe that is what other people think of you, because you have allowed them to put labels on you? You, and only, are in control of your thoughts.

Our thoughts hold so much power! Wherever our thoughts go, our actions follow. So, what path do you want to go down? A path to pure freedom? Or a path to nowhere?

When a negative thought comes into your mind, you can choose to listen to it or choose to say no. We all want freedom. Freedom to be who we want to be, freedom to say what we want to say, and freedom to do what we want to do, but as much as we want freedom, we choose to be prisoners in our own minds. Think about that for a moment.

You have the freedom to be who you really are. It's time to release yourself from your own personal prison. Not sure if that's true for you?

Ask yourself the following:

> ➢ Am I scared to be unapologetically, authentically myself?
> ➢ Do I care what others think?
> ➢ Do I say no to myself?
> ➢ Will this make my _____ (parents, spouse, friends) proud of me?
> ➢ Am I doing what I am truly passionate about?
> ➢ Am I being true to myself?
> ➢ Do you talk yourself out of being who you really are and out of going after your dreams and what you want, because you fear what others might think?
> ➢ Why do you worry so damn much about what others think? Are you living your life for you? Or for someone else?

If you cannot be true to yourself around the people in your life, then maybe it's time to reevaluate your inner circle. The right people who truly love and support you would *never* make you feel uncomfortable for being who you are.

There are people who love us for who they think we can be or for what we might bring to the table, but they don't love you for you! Heck, those types of people are too shallow to even know who the hell you are. You shouldn't have to try so hard to make anyone you love proud, and you need to stop worrying about what anyone else thinks.

There are always people in our lives chirping in our ears about what we need to do, who we need to be, how we need to be, and telling us what they think is best for us. Think about that. How many people do you have like that in your life? How long have they been in your life?

Do the math on that, and figure out how many of those you have. It probably adds up to being a lot of people for a long time. This is just one example that contributes to our limiting beliefs, insecurities, and that negative self-defeating tape that is playing on repeat in your head.

We are all different and unique in our own way. Plus, no two people think alike. If you are a people-pleaser, then this might be tough for you. Not impossible, just tough. The reason is, people-pleasers put a lot of guilt and weight on their own shoulders to make others feel good. That isn't fair. Do yourself a favor, and take all of that weight off of your shoulders! You, my friend, are only responsible for your own weight. Let's not make the load we carry any heavier than it needs to be.

So, what gives? You have to get tired of your own shit! I not only got tired of my own shit but also tired of other people's shit. All of your reactions, choices, and relationships are a reflection of how you feel about yourself. Your environment is a reflection of your self-worth.

Look around at where you are this very moment. Not just aesthetically, but in your job, friendships, relationships, and your health. Do you like what you see and what you have? Do you feel fulfilled? Or are you just going through the motions? Maybe you have a deep, burning knowing inside that you have a much higher calling that you are ignoring. That is the feeling I had for a long time.

I had a negative tape in my head, created from limiting beliefs that were born from experiences as a child and growing up. That limited mindset held me back for way too long.

All the crap you have been through that seemed like a punishment or just bad luck was actually put in front of you to be your teacher, if you allow it to be. Once I allowed all of those painful life experiences to be my teacher, I was able to heal and change that negative tape playing in my head, which had kept me in a box. A boring box I could have never grown in or become the person whom I was meant to be.

If I had listened to the initial thoughts, those insecurities and fears that tried to sneak in, I would never have gone after my dreams. But I didn't listen to those bullshit lies. I *chose* to think differently, that maybe I could or should, and I would! Thank goodness I did, and you are reading this book right now, which means not only did I write it, but it got published!

So, to answer the question, who the hell am I to write this book: I am not a doctor, therapist, or psychologist. I am a woman who has been through hell and back, and who has a deep passion for showing and teaching others how to do the same.

When someone is healed or overcomes adversity or cracks the code on something, you have an unspoken duty: you *must* share and teach others, so they can do the same! Wisdom and growth do not come with age; they come from the lessons learned in the storms. This book was put inside of me to write.

It has always been there, but I only uncovered it once I took my life's adversities as my teachers.

I don't care how old you are, how many kids you have, how much time you don't have, or any other excuses. Stop giving yourself excuses. Stop pointing the finger of blame on everything except yourself. You will only have yourself to blame for staying stuck in a box of mediocrity, living like the characters in the movie, *Groundhog Day*. The theme of that film is how recurrences and repetition are really challenges to change how we do things. You cannot always change everything around you, but you can change your perspective. The one thing we have full control over are our thoughts!

The easiest things to do in life somehow are the hardest. I have yet to figure that out, except to say that maybe we feel, if something is too easy or the solution sounds too simple, it must be hogwash and is just not going to work. We live in a society where people want the magic pill that cures anything overnight, without putting in any effort toward their health. They just want to take a pill and have all their troubles go away. However, when it comes to mental health, people don't even like to discuss it; they just sweep it under the rug. You love magic pills for weight loss, gut health, or the Band-Aids to cover up health problems that require major lifestyle changes… But let's just keep quiet, if you take any medicine for mental health.

Well, I have a pill for you to swallow. Ready? The pill is that you have the power to change, but it is all up to you There is no intensive program for X number of months. All that is required is self-discipline, determination, motivation, and willingness. It is simple, but simple but does not mean easy. It will be difficult at times, but that is where your growth happens. This is why the Universe brings rainy seasons upon us, because there has to be an igniter to your fire that pushes you to become tired of your own shit.

The success of your mindset determines the level of success in every single area of your life!

Your approach to life has been steered by the way you think. So, if your life is not what you want it to be, if it isn't fulfilling and you are not happy, then your approach, which is steered by your thoughts, is clearly not working. Maybe it is time for you to change.

If you are scared of change and how life will be when you finally live your life for yourself, instead of for others, that is okay. It's okay to be scared. In fact, if something scares you a little bit (or a lot), then that is probably what you should be doing!

This Book Was Supposed to Be About...

I knew, as I was fighting Lyme disease (chronic Lyme disease), that I was going to share my story of overcoming Lyme, so others could get well. I couldn't find any stories of hope and healing, when I scoured the Internet for that person who was as sick as I was and then got well. So, I knew I was meant to be the story of hope, inspiration, and beating Lyme!

My first meeting with my publisher, Samantha Joy at Landon Hail Press, was initially about my journey with Lyme. I told her I wanted to share what it was really like, being that sick, living with an invisible disease, being let down by conventional medicine, and finally finding the root cause.

About almost taking my own life and the turning point, when I simply *chose* to believe I could overcome and get well.

I told her the key to me beating chronic Lyme was multifaceted, but there was only one particular thing at the foundation of my healing: my mindset! My *mindset* was the key to every other process being successful in overcoming Chronic Lyme and to my seeing it through.

As Samantha dug deep and asked me questions that I had never been asked or even thought of, it became very apparent that this first book was not just about Lyme. It was about mindset, the ultimate key and weapon for success in every aspect of life!

For ten years, I thought, if I ever had the opportunity to write this book, it would be about Lyme. However, the Universe had something else in store for me. It took the last ten years to unfold, ten years of pain and being lost that ended in the ultimate betrayal, which was a hidden blessing. Within these pages I describe how my life has been unfolding, as I've chosen to shed my old skin and become the person whom I was put on this Earth to be. I had no idea this book was inside of me. It scared the shit out of me, but that is how I knew I needed to write it!

We all go through life, searching for the key to success. We all look at what others do, have, and think; we become yet another sheep in the field instead of being a shepherd. It is time we all stop taking the same approach as someone else, because it worked for them! Stop thinking that, if you can just replicate and do the same things that worked for someone else, then everything in life will fall into place.

Unfortunately, there is not a one-size-fits-all approach to winning the game of life! It just doesn't work that way. Trying to do so will leave you spinning your wheels, which will only lead to unfulfillment and a dead end.

You hold the power in unf*cking yourself, but you give it away. Does your power currently lie in the past, with someone who hurt or wronged you or with a shitty hand you were dealt? If so, then let's get your power back. It is your time to shine!

Before I dive into how my limiting beliefs were created, I will first share what mine were.

- ❖ I was not good enough for anything or anyone.
- ❖ I am not loveable or likable.
- ❖ I am invisible.
- ❖ I deserved everything painful that happened to me. I am just cursed.

It is a little sad for me to write that and reread it in editing, because I would *never, ever* want any of my precious kids to feel that way or to think that way about themselves! I go out of my way to make sure that they don't. The sadness I feel about how I used to think of myself is because I had those thoughts for too long.

What an absolutely miserable way to go through life! Is that what you want for yourself and your loved ones? Imagine what we could all accomplish if we were not living in the past and holding ourselves back! Living in the past does not move you forward. You cannot see what's in front of you if you are looking in the rearview mirror.

It is extremely important to note that you will have your breakthrough at the divine timing set just for you. So, don't for one second think it is too late or worry about whether this should have happened sooner. That is bullshit.

You are the sole creator of your own excuses. Excuses are just a free pass we give ourselves to avoid discomfort. Excuses are just Band-Aids for our insecurities. What are your excuses? Rather, what are your "go-to" excuses? You know, the ones on standby, to get you out of uncomfortable situations you assume the worst of. Be honest with yourself. You must stop looking for excuses in order to take the easy way out and potentially avoid any discomfort.

There will always be some sort of bothersome nuisance in your life or, as I like to say, an emotional vampire. Whether you are healed or unhealed, the annoyances do not go away. emotional vampires and drama queens will always be around. Your perspective and reaction are the only things you can control, and in doing so, you keep your power.

You bring yourself a lot of peace when you have control of your thoughts and what you give your power to. Stop believing every single thought that enters your brain.

When you grow and move up to the next level in your way of thinking, then everything and everyone around you also does. You will outgrow a few of the current people in your life. Who and what you are surrounded with is a reflection of your self-worth.

From this moment forward, be the author of how your story goes, instead of giving everyone else the pen to write it!

It is not going to be all butterflies and roses to break that cycle of self-destruction. To be a butterfly, you have to go through a transformation; a rose has thorns all the way to its beautiful petals. Stop denying the thought that, with age, you have outgrown past hurts or trauma. There is no outgrowing or running away from any hurt, pain, or anger. You have to address all of it in order to heal, so you can cut those invisible chains holding you back.

So, grab your shovel and put your boots on, because shit is about to get *deep!* It is time to get rid of what is not serving you well, surrender to letting go, while embracing what can be.

You hold the key to your freedom. Freedom in your mind, freedom from the past, and freedom to be unapologetically and authentically yourself.

*****

Takeaway: *Time goes by no matter what! You can either look back and be really happy you did something, or you can look back and wish you had done it. Only one of those decisions will you regret!*

So, who the fuck are you?

CHAPTER 2

Break Out of the Safety Box

You can only go as high as the ceiling above you so stop putting limits on yourself. Get rid of the ceiling and walls, so you can spread your wings and fly!

I WAS SITTING BY the warm fire with my blanket, cuddled up with my family and our black Lab, Charlotte May. I felt safe and secure. Everything I loved and all that I needed was right there with me. I was 100% content, happy, and at peace. My three kids were content; I looked at them in admiration of who they are and what they will become. I reflected on how my life was and who I was, when I once lived in my "safety box." I would never be where I am today, if I had not broken out of that box.

What is the safety box? This invisible cage is built by our own fears, insecurities, and those of others that we allow to enclose us. It is made up of walls and a ceiling of confinement created by our limiting beliefs. But why?

We put ourselves in this invisible "safe haven" to protect us from being hurt and having an experience similar to the ones from our past that still wound us. But there is another reason for our having this safety box: we are absolutely terrified of the unknown. We are scared shitless of being uncomfortable and taking a chance on ourselves. The thing is, when you put a ceiling above yourself, then you put a cap on your potential. Always have a floor—those are your boundaries. But take the walls and ceiling down, so you can spread your wings and fly.

I was forty-one years old. I felt safe and secure because I was home with all that I cherished and dearly loved. However, it wasn't just the material things in my environment that made me feel protected and shielded. I am extremely grateful for those things that protect me, yes, but I refer to an internal mental feeling outside of those external factors. This feeling was very different. I was genuinely happy, content, and at peace with who I am and everything that made me who I am. I felt a deep knowing of extreme gratitude, understanding, and appreciation of my transformation and growth. I had created my own happiness, freedom, confidence, and self-love. No one can ever take that from me.

It wasn't always this way for me.

There was a time when that scenario I describe was just a temporary, short-lived sense of happiness. It was based on only external factors, things that could be disrupted at any moment and gone. I was not content with my life for almost forty years. I never before had had true happiness. There were fleeting moments when I'd felt temporary happiness or joy, but only if every little detail fit my image of perfection without any objections. I most certainly was never content. I could have an amazing day, but the happy feelings were fleeting.

You cannot be content when you just accept life the way it is. Acceptance is not contentment, and there is no settling in contentment. Deep-down inside, you can feel you are meant for so much more! You are merely going through the motions every day, while ignoring the fire of your purpose, which burns within us all.

Contentment cannot be achieved without self-love, approval, and acceptance. Once you create happiness within yourself, after healing your limited mindset, and are 100% unapologetically, authentically *you, then and only then can you be truly content*!

Feeling safe and secure no longer requires a safety box and is no longer tangible; rather, it is an internal knowing and environment in which I am freely, authentically me, surrounded by those who unconditionally love me, and through all the different seasons that may come my way, rain or shine.

Are you relying on external factors to make you safe and secure? Ask yourself these questions:

- Are you uncomfortable being your authentic self no matter who you are around?
- Are you careful not to rock the boat in order to keep the peace at home or in your job?
- Do you make choices based on others' ideas and opinions so that you are approved of?
- Do you make choices based on achieving or maintaining a certain social status?

If you answered yes to just one of those questions, then you are relying solely on external factors to make you feel safe and secure. That is not going to make you feel content!

How do you know if you are ready for growth? When you become uncomfortable with your current situation, behaviors, insecurities, and lack of purpose, then you are ready! Being comfortable is *not* an ingredient for growth.

You have no one to blame for the box you have put yourself in and allowed others to put you in. You set boundaries for what you allow from others without even realizing you are. That box is simply the "comfort zone" for you and others. People crave comfort! We all want to feel secure and protected, whether physically or emotionally.

Anything outside of the box is the unknown and scary. If you veer outside of the comfort zones you have allowed others to put in place for you, that is threatening to them; they fear what you might do, learn, or become.

Your growth will shine a light on others' insecurities.

When you mix all of your insecurities with your partner's and that of those closest to you, then you are in one tight box. Growth cannot happen when there is no room for it.

Guess what? You can make room for growth by breaking every one of those walls down! How freeing does that sound? Stop worrying about who you will let down or what will be disrupted, because you are only letting yourself down. Never again will I live in a box I created to keep me safe, and I will never again live in someone else's box, just to keep them comfortable.

It is in the discomfort, however, that you grow. But the unknown can be scary. Answer this: which is scarier? Venturing out into the unknown you know nothing about? Or staying safe in your comfy little box but never experiencing the life you were meant to live?

I know how terrifying it was to leave the comfort zone and go after my dreams. There was no promise, no guarantee that I would succeed. I had no clue what to do, and I did not know one person who could help me break into the new world I sought. So, I shifted my mindset. At that point, I had done a lot of healing and was able to shift my mindset to one that benefited me.

I realized I was choosing to believe in the fears of failure, which was holding me back, so just as much as I was giving the negative thoughts the power and energy, I could shift that to thinking positive about my desires. I remember thinking I had lived long enough only listening to the negative. Where had that got me? I knew the conclusion on that view, but what about if I chose to believe? There is only one way to find out!

There are only so many fish you can catch at the surface, and not a lot of variety. You are going to have to go out in that scary ocean, if you want a bigger fish.

It isn't easy to look into our own lives from the outside, and appraise it without being defensive. Accepting and acknowledging our own faults and flaws is a hard pill to swallow. You are so accustomed to pointing a finger at anything or anyone else as the cause, so when you decide to no longer do that, the only place you have to point to is, well, right in the mirror.

Something special happens when we hear other people's stories of hardships and how they overcome them, let them reflect into our own life, and give hope. You can then recognize some of the same patterns in your own life. Hearing another's journey and about their transformation into their true self ignites our own self-awareness, which allows us to see ourselves from the outside looking in. The same discomfort and maybe even embarrassment that you feel from your own wounds are easier to face after you hear about another person's struggles. We always think we are alone in the darkness, but we never are.

The moment we were born, we quickly became acclimated to our environment, based on what created comfort, security, warmth, and nourishment for us, and at what levels we received them. This sense of security is carried with us, as we grow up. It affects how we behave, how we respond, and what we need to stay safe and secure.

We all grow up in a bubble, only knowing life one way. We assume the way of life we are accustomed to is the same for everyone. As we grow up, our bubble pops. We realize that other people live differently and our bubbles is.... just a bubble.

The money, the house, the clothes, how much food, what neighborhood—none of that really matters. Those "things" do not create happiness. So, regardless of the material items you grew up with, none of those external things stop the "happening" of limiting beliefs, triggers, and insecurities. All that is created from the external factors is an outward appearance of your life, where you seem to be happy, well put together, and successful. Frankly, too many people live their lives to impress others. That has to get tiring!

Let's get started on finding the pieces to the puzzle of why you have the limited beliefs you have. It begins with what created a sense of safety for your growing up. There is no wrong answer here.

For example, as a child, my sense of safety involved being home with my family, my routine, and not getting in trouble. I did not like to upset anyone. I paid close attention to what my siblings did that irritated my parents and took notes on what not to do and what worked.

I hated it when there was strife or conflict in the house. I didn't like it when my brothers wrestled or argued or when my parents disagreed. I have always been inquisitive, analytical, and opinionated. I never felt anything other than different from my family.

As a child, you quickly go from the innocent state of mind of an infant to discovering what makes you not cry. What makes you not feel scared or lonely or like you have upset someone. You learn what to do to receive praise, and you learn what creates disappointment. My point is, during our childhood, that environment and the experiences we go through create limiting beliefs, mindset, and insecurities, and they dictate what we need to feel seen and heard.

Ask yourself these questions:

- ❖ What made you feel safe as a child?
- ❖ What made you feel safe as a teenager/young adult?
- ❖ What makes you feel safe now?

As a child, feeling safe typically consists of the basic comforts, like being fed, warm, and clean, and receiving affection. As we grow up, there are additions to what makes us feel safe. As a teenager, fitting in and not being made fun of are added. As an adult, being financially stable and your accomplishments are then tacked on.

In those examples, the needs of a child are pure and simple. As we grow up, all the other additional things we need to feel safe stem from various limiting beliefs that slowly creep into our minds. At such a young age, we begin to strive constantly to *prove* ourselves to others.

Judging Others is Your Defense Mechanism

Who gave you a gavel to judge? While you sit in a restaurant, waiting for your food and looking at everyone walking by or sitting around you, you constantly make assumptions. Is what you are doing simply observing? Or are you judging? Not sure?

Observing is simply looking and perceiving. Judging is when you assume how someone is—how they live, their personality, and maybe even what they stand for. I am extremely observant and always have been, but I also was once very judgmental.

How we behave and interact in public, along with our thought processes, all are formed from the environment we grew up in. Watching how our family interacts and communicates as we grow up greatly affects how we will, as well. We are truly products of our environment. However, when we grow up, we then can choose either to stay the same or to change.

When everyone around you behaves and thinks in a certain way, it can become a crutch for you to not change. It is easier to stay the same and be like everyone around us than to change. For what will people think?

When I got tired of my own shit, I began to really work on myself internally. There are so many different layers to uncover and heal. They are not pretty, so make sure the regret you feel as get to each layer never sticks with you.

Regret robs you of freedom and happiness. I say that because I felt a lot of regret when I realized how judgmental I had been up until that moment. The thing is, many times, you know how you are, but the second you think about it, that thought is quickly followed with an excuse, and you give yourself a free pass to keep acting the same way.

Be honest with yourself, and do not attach an excuse to it, just so you can continue to ignore it.

The moment you stop giving yourself excuses is the moment you make yourself pliable for change. Excuses are a roadblock that keeps you stuck. Observing life, people, and our surroundings is perfectly normal. Just make sure your observations are without criticisms, assumptions, and judgments. Living with an invisible disease comes with a lot of criticism. When I was very sick with Lyme disease, no one could *see* that I was sick. My symptoms of hell were not visible. People just thought I was complaining and overreacting. Think of how many times you have been wrong with your assumptions?

Never judge a book by its cover, for you do not know the contents within.

You must stop looking to others and to material things to bring you comfort and fill your voids. (Maybe you don't even think what I am saying is correct or applies to your life; but I believe, if you are holding this book, you know deep-down there are invisible obstacles blocking you from your true potential.)

I was mind-blown when I put my own puzzle together. It was hard sometimes, putting the pieces together, but it was much harder living my life not being true to myself.

I encourage you to journal as you finish each chapter. Write down *all* that you feel when ideas and things are stirred up; do not ignore anything. These may include memories, feelings, fears, or insecurities. This is the beginning of finding out your limiting beliefs and their root cause.

Truth is that the safety box is nothing more than a cage we created ourselves to protect us from fears formed by the root of our limiting beliefs. However, it truly offers us no protection. Rather, it becomes a prison for our pain. And in the same ways as it was *you* who created your safety box, so it is also you who has to break it down and free yourself.

If you want to unlock your true potential and live a life with limitless possibilities, then you have to take the limits off of yourself. It all begins with your mindset.

*****

Aren't you ready to free yourself, break out of your personal prison, and live your fucking life on your terms?

CHAPTER 3

The Birth of My Limiting Beliefs

We don't get to choose the seed of our limiting beliefs, but we do have the choice about how long we water it and allow it to be a weed in our life.

HEALING IS CONSTANT, with many different layers. I always assumed, once you healed, that was it. But I discovered on my own journey what healing really looks like and how it feels. I compare it to peeling an onion: there is layer after layer, and just when you think you have reached the last layer, there is another.

Triggers from your past still get your attention, but the effect on you is different. You recognize them through a different lens, like from the outside looking in. This does not mean you do not get bothered by certain triggers that once greatly affected your life in a negative way. I mean it is more of an irritation and no longer a wound.

Let's face it: all of the crap from our past creates the determining factors to where you set boundaries. Nothing goes away, but it changes your mindset to one that no longer allows the ghosts from the past to haunt you.

I never thought I would be sharing the most heart-wrenching and unpleasant memories I have ever endured. There was a time when I prayed that they would stay buried. None of us want anyone else knowing what pains we have experienced. It is embarrassing even to think about; we fear others will think we are crazy. What is funny is that I no longer have that thought, which is all fear. I am not ashamed of my past, nor should you be. For me, that realization was just another sign of how much I have overcome and healed.

I am not going to gloss over key moments in my childhood and teenage years that were either the seeds or results of my wounded mindset. That is not fair to you, my reader. I cannot ask you to dig up the ugly stuff if I do not do the same.

No one wants to dig up ghosts from their past, but those ghosts will continue to haunt you until you put them to rest. You must find the weapon that created the wounds, or they will continue to bleed on every part of your life.

Going through life while putting a Band-Aid on a bullet wound in the form of alcohol, drugs, overworking, food, technology, binge-watching, and over-scheduling, just to numb yourself and block the pain, is no way to live. *You cannot heal from what you won't feel to deal with.* Period.

Is facing your demons and the pain of your past absolutely necessary for this process? 100%. Are you going to have to face anyone who hurt you? No. You just have to face the memory and feelings you experienced, which will show you the limiting belief that was born from that pain.

Maybe you even have a good relationship with that person today or have forgiven them. You still have to revisit every catalyst that planted the seed, since that is the root cause of that particular limiting belief, which has been a weight in your life for far too long. We are going to pull the weeds out one by one!

So, how were these beliefs and insecurities created? Every single experience from the second you are born, including the environment you grew up in and the behavior of every single person you lived and interacted with, on top of all that you are exposed to in life, these all together created and shaped your limiting mindset and insecurities. For example, I grew up in a very critical negative household, so I had the limiting belief that I was not good enough and that nothing would ever work out for me.

You only need to confront yourself and the painful memories. This process is for you, about you, and no one else! Truth is, the ones who hurt us emotionally were the root-cause to a limiting belief, but *they* have no idea. Their reactions and behavior stemmed from their very own limited mindset and unhealed wounds. There is a good chance they have no idea of their part in your insecurities.

This is not a blame game. In fact, getting rid of a victim mindset is one of the many invisible chains we are going to cut. You cannot live your life worrying about what others think. Anyone who is offended or feels it is about them is reacting from their own insecurities. You are only responsible for healing your insecurities, not theirs. Defensive people are merely people who are constantly reacting from unhealed trauma and insecurities.

I know this because that used to be me. I believed every little thing that someone said or did was targeted at me. Once I did the work and cut all of those invisible chains, I was no longer offended by so darn much! What's funny is, when you heal, you clearly see when someone else hasn't, even if you just met!

A healed person communicates very differently, and it is not possible to have certain realizations when you are unhealed. The communication and understanding are on another level. So, I no longer care who knows the truth about me or any part of my life, because I know the truth, and it is unimportant if anyone else does. Look, trying to always "prove your point" is f*cking exhausting. Frankly, there shouldn't be anyone in your life whom you feel that way with.

Here is a really good example. People ask me, "Aren't you worried about what your family will think or feel, if you are sharing personal details that they were involved in?" And my answer is, "No."

Did I think about that for a fleeting moment? Absolutely. However, this book is about how limiting beliefs are born, so sharing the cause and effect is absolutely necessary. Holding those parts back would completely eliminate my ability to teach you. It is in reading about my root causes that you will have the ability to reflect and find our own root causes.

There is no blame on my parents or anyone from my past for any of their *behaviors* that created wounds or contributed to the limited mindset I once had. I believe my parents did the very best they could, raising me and my three siblings. They parented based on their own childhood and life experiences. Any and all of their unhealed wounds and limiting beliefs were passed down through their parenting.

I did the very same with my kids, until I shattered my own limiting beliefs. Once I did, I then was able to mother my kids in a completely different way. That is the best gift I could have ever given them. I did not want to pass down my unhealed wounds to my kids. We must stop doing that! You either parent from a healed mindset or from an unhealed one. So, which mindset do you want to teach, love, and live from?

I have a lot of great memories from growing up, but the "good stuff" is not what I detail here. That is important to remember. You do not need to grow up in an abusive, destructive environment to have wounds and limiting beliefs. When I hear people say that certain behaviors they were around, growing up, are normal and just part of life, all I really hear is an excuse as to why they should not do things any differently. Most people have no idea their behavior has ever left such an impact on others' lives. My parents were not doing anything on purpose to try to create a specific way of thinking or insecurity for me. No one can address anything they are not even aware of! Until an issue is brought to someone's attention, how could they ever realize there was an issue?

No one is responsible for another's actions, only for their own. At the same time, it is absolutely okay to voice and share how another's actions have hurt us and impacted our lives, whether in a positive way or a negative way. It doesn't make much sense for anyone who has ever hurt us or wronged us, intentionally or not, to get upset for someone voicing that experience.

To the people who say, "How dare you tell the world your personal pain and make me look bad!" *Well, how could I not share all that I went through and learned from, so others could do the same?* Not to would be selfish.

My childhood was "normal," in the sense of what normal looked like for me. There is no one definition of "normal." Normal is simply what is normal for you, regardless of what it is for someone else. As kids growing up, we are very naïve. You just assume that everyone else lives a similar life in a similar environment. All you know, growing up, is based on what you are exposed to.

This means all the emotions, communication, interactions, love, affection, expectations, and discipline you were around. But that is not all! Combine all of that with how you, specifically, process information, learn, react, and respond, including your emotions and emotional needs! We are all uniquely different. No two people are wired the same way.

Growing Up

I am the youngest of four, with my sister being the oldest and two brothers in between us. My sister is nine years older than me, so I spent more time with my brothers and was a girly-girl tomboy. Both of my parents were self-employed and worked really hard to provide for our large family, making sure we always had what we needed.

My parents grew up with parents who instilled a work-hard ethic, just as ours did for me and my siblings. We didn't venture out a whole lot, always staying pretty close to home and in our comfort zone.

We saw our extended family a good bit, especially around the holidays. I was a quiet, reserved kid, until I felt comfortable around who was there. I was always observing and analyzing people and my environment, and I was sensitive to the energy around me.

It was very easy to see that people from both sides of the family had favorites. I experienced being a favorite on one side and not a favorite on the other side. It was never pointed out to me, I just knew. As a mom of three, I cannot even begin to understand how anyone could play favorites with their kids or grandkids.

Growing up, I felt different from those around me, which made me shy. To my young mind, all other kids communicated and played so easily together, and I never felt like I fit in. In fact, I struggled for a very long time with feeling different. As a kid, you just want to fit in. I began to view myself in a negative way. I just wanted to belong and be liked. I wanted to feel accepted and good enough. My limiting belief of not feeling good enough was just beginning here.

How do those feelings become a need or desire inside an innocent mind? Your environment, mixed with how you internalize, react, and respond.

What happened that made me think that way or need to fit in? I constantly observed the criticism and judging that occurred in my household. It was a bit of a negative environment, always more "the glass is half empty." Both of my parents grew up in a very similar environment, where there was judging, criticizing, comparison, and pointing the finger.

It is hard to see that your mindset might be limited. That is why some never change. The moment you stop learning and being open to ideas, whenever you believe you know everything, that is the moment you stop growing. Don't sell yourself short. I will still be learning until the day I take my last breath.

How about you? Is it hard for you to learn new ideas and ways of thinking, because it makes you uncomfortable? Pay attention to what makes you uncomfortable, because there is a good chance there is something the Universe is trying to show and teach you.

The way of thinking I grew up around was very closed-minded, simply because that was passed down. I felt like there was more questioning than understanding. More talking and less listening.

I have always been very inquisitive, and that means I typically have a lot of questions. I just want to understand everything. To some that can come off as annoying or like you are questioning them, but you are just trying to understand and learn. That was difficult for me, because my parents' favorite answer was *no*. I always replied with, "*Why?*" which was often followed by, "Just 'cause..."

So again, I would ask, "But why?" Until it was made clear I needed to stop asking, because that's as far as it would go. Not knowing the why always left me frustrated, and it still does, but now I understand it is okay if we don't have an answer.

As a mom, I now realize that kids just want to understand everything! The world is new to them, their brains are growing fast, and they just want to learn and make sense of their world.

So, the more curiosity you leave unanswered for your kids growing up, the more answers they will search for, the more things they try to figure out themselves.

I now believe kids should be curious, so they can use their imagination, as they should. It is our job, as parents, to teach them and guide them. Why do so many parents want to take away kids' imaginations and make them feel dumb for dreaming big? Honestly, it wouldn't hurt more adults to use theirs.

My parents loved us, and I have a lot of great memories, so I will never take any of that away. But what sticks with me, and what as a child I always sought after, is approval! Every single one of us wants to feel understood by our parents and loved ones. It doesn't mean you agree with or even feel the same way. It just means you understand the way someone thinks, feels, and needs.

All three of my kids are different from one another, and I understand each of them. (At least, I do my very best!) None of us think alike, and that is okay!

That brings me to the fact that I did not feel understood by my family, growing up. It felt more like, "Here is a box, and you need to fit in the box." Anything outside of the box was bad and never an option. I don't fit in a box really well. Who does?

My parents did not like to be challenged or questioned, which made me feel frustrated and lonely. As I grew up, I questioned more things and ideas. I badly needed to spread my wings to fly, but that is kind of hard to do in a box.

I longed to be understood and seen. My sister was nine years older than me, so she moved out when I was nine years old. My two older brothers didn't really want to hang out with their little sister, so I often felt alone. I still didn't stop asking them to play with me, because I always had hope that they would give in. Not very often. In fact, I didn't really make a lot of close friends until third grade. I was shy and just wanted to be liked and have a friend. I didn't want to be told *no*, that someone didn't want to play with me.

As you see, at a very young age, all I wanted and needed was to feel seen and understood. For the longest time, I wanted to feel accepted. Like I wasn't the bother my siblings made me feel. They didn't do it on purpose. They just didn't know.

I cannot remember a time when my mom wasn't on a diet. I learned to associate guilt with food by watching my mom feel guilty and ashamed for the slightest indulgence. She would hide a Snickers bar wrapper in her Diet Coke can. She couldn't eat anything without scrutiny. I hated it. I would often defend my mom or beg her to defend herself, but she never would. Instead, my mom put up with it because it was easier, and in doing so, that kept the peace.

Apparently, keeping the peace has nothing to do with your inner peace.

At a very young age, I observed being thin and having overall good looks as important and necessary things, associated with being approved of and noticed. In sharing this part of my upbringing, it makes the mindset I had of the association of physical appearance with approval and acceptance very easy to understand.

So, what downward spiral effect did that have on me? *Let's see...*

I started exercising on the treadmill and weighing myself when I was eleven years old. I suffered from my first two eating disorders at age twelve: anorexia and bulimia.

My God, you are thinking, how did her parents not know? Not sure, but they didn't. I would weigh myself daily, sometimes multiple times. I was obsessed with my weight. I did not feel skinny enough, and I hated the dimples I would get on my thighs, when I sat cross-legged. I hated my nose and thought it looked like a ski slope, so I would push the tip of my nose down anytime I could and hold it in place, hoping it would eventually stay down.

Is it easy for you to see how this limiting belief developed in me, as a child? Children do not know any better. As a child growing up, as teenager or young adult, and even as I grew into a grown woman, I struggled with picking my looks apart! It makes me extremely sad to think about my precious daughter ever being that way to herself!

Not one single person was aware of the constant struggle I had with my body. My mom never knew, even though I knew about hers. What's more, my seeing her struggle and seeing her be critiqued for her weight are what birthed my limiting belief.

Any limiting beliefs that a parent has that remain unhealed are passed down to their kids.

I did not feel comfortable in my own body. I picked myself apart and critiqued myself to no end. At twelve years old, when my first period came, I had no idea what was happening with my body! Puberty and periods had never been explained. That was a super-awkward time, which it is anyway, but especially when you are not really expecting it and have no idea what is going on.

The fact I already felt so uncomfortable in my own body made going through puberty hell. When junior high started, I felt really awkward! I had naturally curly hair that I hid, and even my own mother did not know. I am sure you are wondering how I hid this from my own mom... I would blow-dry my hair as soon as I got out of the shower. I was terrified of my peers knowing I had naturally curly hair and then making fun of me by calling me a poodle. I had witnessed those same kids do that to anyone who had naturally curly hair. Of course, when my mom found out, she made me wear my hair to school in all its naturally curly glory! Lovely.

By thirteen years old, I never felt like I was pretty, good enough, capable, or seen. I felt invisible. Being a teenager is awkward enough as it is. When puberty starts, the new hormones just add to the discomfort. When you mix in a combination of emotional turmoil with the heightened emotions in a teenager, that can lead to trouble.

All the limiting beliefs that formed in my mind created a negative, self-defeating tape that played on repeat in my head, fueling my insecurities and reinforcing my belief that they were all true.

*****

This is how my limiting beliefs were born, including some of their ripple effects in my life. The yearning I had to know I was good enough was so strong, it led me down a path where I stopped at nothing to feel seen and good enough. That unhealthy path had very unhealthy consequences.

CHAPTER 4

The Fire of Sadness Blew Up in Flames

When pressure builds up with no release, then combustion is without fail.

I WAS SCREAMING FOR ATTENTION. Being a teenager can be a really lonely, awkward time. It most certainly was for me. I really wanted to feel approved of and not feel shame for how I felt inside. The sadness I felt inside grew like a wildfire, and I felt so ashamed for not feeling "normal," it made the pain inside me worse.

My parents were not approachable, and the fear I had inside of telling them what I was feeling was terrifying, so I just kept it all inside. The problem with that is, when you bury pain and hide it, it comes out in other ways, and it isn't always pretty.

I started cutting myself with razors on my upper thigh when I was twelve, just to feel the pain. In my naïve, immature mind, *I thought making myself feel pain would heal mine.* It was also my way of calling for help. I did not realize that at the time, but that's exactly what I was doing! I was *crying* for help! I felt so invisible, I was really acting out just to see if someone would notice.

I cut myself for about a year. It took my mom almost a year to find the cuts. She, of course, was shocked, as any parent would be, and upset. Seeing her reaction of anger, which was really probably more painful than anything, upset me even more. It was fuel on the fire. All I wanted to see was her care, for her to see my cry for help, to see my pain. I wanted her to hold me and tell me she loved me and that I was good enough.

My naïve mind truly thought she would wake up and see how I had been hurting and feeling, and why. I wanted my mom to fix the pain and sadness that was inside of me and make it all go away! I truly felt my mom could read my mind! So, when my mom "ignored" my cries for help, I thought she was doing it on purpose, in a way. That made everything else I was feeling worse.

When you are young, you think your parents can fix everything. Just push the magic button, and all is well.

My mom's reaction was more of "what were you thinking?" and rightfully so. She could not relate to what I was doing or why, since she'd never experienced what I had. As a mom, I would say the same, but because of what I have been through, I understand the cries for help. My mom could not, since she'd never experienced anything like this in her own life.

Experience provides insight and wisdom. It is like being able to see into another life through a clear glass versus a frosted glass. Parents, when your kids are acting up and are triggered easily, that is a good indicator that there is something else going on. That is why it is imperative that our kids know they can always talk to us.

I felt I tried so many ways to get my parents to notice me. I would think to myself, "They must not care enough to even notice I am not eating, that I'm obsessed with my weight, cutting, over-exercising, hate everything about me. They don't notice me making remarks they would be better off without me."

Were any of those self-defeating thoughts true? Did my parents really not care? Absolutely not! Being a thirteen-year-old girl, who had to figure out periods and deal with hormones, along with feeling invisible and carrying the weight of shame, was a lot to deal with. Escaping the pain of all that turmoil inside me was all I wanted. I couldn't stand feeling like that for another second.

The fire of sadness had grown so much inside of me, *all* I could think about was *making it go away*. I did not truly grasp the concept of "suicide." Stopping the emotional pain was all I wanted. I did not possess the tools necessary to properly deal with what I was going through.

Times were very different in the nineties. It was 1994, to be exact. Mental health is still a tough concept for people to grasp, but it was especially tough back then.

One night, as I was talking to one of my best friends on the phone, I told him I had taken a bunch of pills. I said that I was sorry, but I couldn't take it anymore. Soon after, I was borderline unconscious.

Thankfully, he called my parents' phone and told my mom he was really scared about what I had done, afraid he might lose me. My parents ran to my room, screaming and terrified. I could barely verify the horrific truth.

I clearly wasn't thinking. I was just a child, wanting and needing approval. I yearned so desperately to just feel seen and be told I was more than enough. I made a really dumb decision. A teenager's brain, a child's brain, does not think and function the way an adult brain does. As parents, we often forget that.

My mom got me in her Suburban and rushed me to the hospital. She was crying and yelling the whole way. Not yelling out of anger, but because she was scared and in shock. That was when I vaguely realized, through my foggy brain, what I had really done.

I didn't like seeing my mom so sad and upset. That was never my intention. My intention was to stop my hurt, not cause it. I felt like being alive and on Earth was more of a burden. I truly believed no one would notice.

The night was a blur. At the ER, they pumped my stomach and hooked me up to an IV, and I was saved. In order to be released, a psychiatrist or psychotherapist has to evaluate you and determine you are no longer at risk. My mom's mom, my grandmother, was a psychotherapist.

My grandmother and I were not close at the time. She had her favorites, and I was never one of them, which I knew full well. She made sure to let me know she was doing my mom a favor and how I was embarrassing her. I was not surprised by any of it but what I noticed and will never understand was that she was stone-cold. She did not have one ounce of sadness or fear for my health at all.

To top it off, her career and her passion were supposed to be helping those in a deep, dark place. She helped people to overcome these things! I was her granddaughter, her own blood, and she couldn't have cared less. It couldn't have been more obvious.

I stayed quiet on the way home, listening as my parents berated me for what I had attempted. They never once asked why or cared about what could have possibly gotten me to that point. I realized they didn't understand, because they didn't try to. It scared the shit out of them, but I felt like I had just embarrassed them.

I became numb. I pushed down all the pain and sadness. I told myself it obviously did not matter, and if an attempted suicide did not make my parents notice me and make me feel good enough to try for their approval, it all seemed useless. I decided, when I turned eighteen, I would be on my own and my own damn boss.

I was done seeking approval from my parents, so I just stopped trying. I resented their lack of understanding. I felt I would never get it from them. The desire I had to seek their approval turned into a bottomless void that I would continue trying to fill.

False Confidence

Numb. I became numb once I came home from the hospital. I also felt shame, embarrassment, stupidity, and more invisible than ever. I hated being home, because after that, it felt like my parents and siblings judged me. I felt they looked down on me for what I'd done. They didn't understand. Not one of them ever tried to just talk to me, to see why I'd done that or said they were happy I wasn't successful. Those were the thoughts that flooded my teenage mind.

My parents became even more strict on me, making me feel even more trapped. I knew it was because they didn't trust me, all of which made me feel more alienated.

Like I said earlier, junior high, with all the physical and emotional changes we're experiencing, was just flat-out an awkward time for me. I try to stay cognizant of this, now that my oldest two are teenagers. I want my kids to feel confident inside and out, just like I wanted to, as a teen. Confidence wasn't really talked about much in the nineties. It was more of a perception of someone who looked good, was talented or athletic, and in just how they carried themselves. Truth is, that was probably mostly what I call false confidence.

Feeling confident in who you are from the inside out changes how you approach every aspect of life. *False confidence* is being confident in an ability you possess, an activity you excel at, or your physical appearance, but you lack confidence internally with who you are.

You have to perform, show your talent, or receive recognition in order to feel confident. We should all feel confident in our abilities, as each and every one of us is talented. Having *internal* confidence is a game changer. There will always be someone more talented or prettier, but nothing can take internal confidence away. True confidence does not need any external validation or approval. It can only be obtained by you approving, loving, and accepting yourself unconditionally.

Junior high, for me, was the beginning of extra-curricular activities where you truly competed. I'd started playing the violin in elementary school, so I joined the orchestra in junior high. I also joined the tennis team. My mom and brothers played tennis, so our family as a whole would sometimes practice together. I was really good at both violin and tennis, so as rankings and competitions began, my confidence grew. False confidence, by my terms today, but I felt confident for the first time ever.

Making good grades was easy for me, and I always strived for straight As. I began to focus on what I was good at and my achievements. In some ways, looking back, I was numbing myself and trying to fill voids through my achievements.

When we have confidence, we carry ourselves differently, we perform differently, we choose differently, and we feel differently, too. You put yourself on a different wavelength of attraction, when you exude true inner confidence.

Once we find our talents and what we are good at, we then practice and practice so we continue to improve and get better. There is excitement we have, knowing where our strengths lie.

Take that same disciplined mentality, practicing, and practice on improving your mindset. Will it be easy at first? No! There will be discomfort within the growing pains. Some days, you will feel you went two steps backward instead of forward, but it is like that with anything you are working on to improve and becoming better at.

This analogy, of comparing the growth you experience when improving an external trait to improving your mindset, is a simple hack to help you stay on track as you level up. Consistency creates confidence, as in the more you do a particular thing, the better you get.

You must embrace your authentic self, by staying in the present without regretting a part of your past that you cannot change. Accept yourself where you are in the moment—emotionally, mentally, and physically. Stop wishing you had more or looked different. Instead, take action on creating the life and body you desire. Stop giving any of your energy to self-defeating thoughts that are not even true. Start giving yourself grace, compassion, and patience.

Naïve and Deceived

By ninth grade, I no longer felt so awkward in my teenage body, which was used to dealing with all the fun teenage stuff our bodies go through. I began high school as a sophomore, which is how high school was where I grew up. I immediately made varsity on the tennis team. I was the youngest player and didn't know anyone. All of my friends were JV or not playing tennis.

I had a late birthday, so I was always the youngest in my grade. I was fourteen for the first week of my sophomore year. I drew a lot of attention from the older boys. I wasn't much of a dater, mainly because my parents were super-strict, and asking to do anything outside of school just wasn't worth it.

There was one senior boy who really liked me. He asked me out a few times, but I told him *no* the first few times. He wouldn't take no for an answer. He asked my friends for my phone number and eventually got it. (This is back when we had house phones with cords connecting it to the wall!) There was no caller ID, so one night, when the phone rang and I answered, it was him.

I was embarrassed, because I'd told him *no* so many times. He was nice and flattering. He made me feel pretty and wanted, and I liked it. He was eighteen, and I had just turned fifteen. I somehow got my parents to let me date him and that became my first serious relationship. But it was not healthy. In fact, it was absolutely toxic.

The void of not feeling approved of, seen, and loved was desperate. When you are desperate to fill emotional voids, you look past any and all flaws that should be major red flags. That is exactly what I did. I overlooked toxicity and abuse, because I was so desperate to fill my voids.

It is easy to see why that relationship happened, isn't it? The need to feel accepted, approved, and loved was stronger than my care for self-respect. It was like a chase. I was chasing after a constant moving goal post. No matter what disrespect he meted out, I just kept on chasing.

All of the flattery he used initially, to win me over, completely stopped once I was his. He stopped making me feel special.

I was so young, though, I didn't realize what I had gotten myself into. I didn't know and understand the things I know now. I didn't have any wisdom then. I was a naïve teenager who thought I could handle it all on my own. About a year later, I learned he liked to drink. A lot. I wasn't even twenty-one years old at the time. Some days, he would drink excessively; on those days, I would not be able to get ahold of him. I would be scared that something might have happened to him.

I might not hear from him for two or three days, sometimes, and I felt so upset and hurt. But no matter what he did, I stayed with him. He did what he wanted to do, and I also put up with it. His behavior toward me when he was drinking became emotionally abusive, especially if I was ever upset about his drinking.

The person I am today would never even be around someone who behaves that way.

Five years later, when I was just twenty years old, we got married. I knew it was a bad decision in my gut, but not only did I ignore that, I was naïve enough to believe he would change. Where did my idea that marriage changes a couple's relationship come from? Marriage does not change a relationship, nor should it. The reason a couple decides to marry in the first place is that they are happy, in love, and bring out the best in each other. At least that's how it should be. Marriage will not fix any problems or make someone a better person. We must stop thinking that it will.

I had no business getting married, and honestly, I don't even think I quite understood marriage. I cannot even fathom the idea of one of my kids getting married or even wanting to at twenty years old! I was clearly not thinking. I was so stubborn and hellbent that no one would tell me what to do. I think I was particularly determined to prove I could do exactly what I wanted to do. I actually believed he loved me and that it would all work out. As you can imagine, it didn't. That marriage was a disaster waiting to happen. It quickly blew up in flames.

As soon as we were married, I realized he was an alcoholic. His drinking got way worse, as well as his benders. Since I had a false belief that marriage would somehow make him stop drinking, his staying gone, and being mean, the hurt I felt each time he did these things got worse.

I would cry to him about his behavior, telling him how it made me feel, hoping he would see what his actions were doing to me. He let me know that was a bad idea and to keep my mouth shut. The emotional abuse became worse, and then he became physically and sexually abusive.

I was living in pure hell. I was terrified of him. Everything I did or said was questioned. If any guy I knew through work ever said hi to me in public, I paid for it. I became quiet. I would work as late as I could at the optical shop, where I was an optician, to avoid ever going home to our apartment. I took college classes, which, due to my work schedule, were mostly at night. I tried to be gone and away from him as much as possible.

I no longer cared about his benders; they brought me peace, knowing I was safe for at least a few days. I became really quiet around him, afraid to say the wrong thing. That only helped me temporarily, as my silence began to infuriate him, too, and my struggle not to say the wrong thing was apparent.

I was also afraid to tell anyone. Anyone who has not experienced being in an abusive situation always wonders why the victim never says anything. The reason is because, not only do you think no one will believe you, but also what will happen, if the abuser finds out. I was just waiting for the right moment when I could leave. I lived in fear of what he would do every single day. I was ashamed. My body felt like a garbage can.

One night, after he was so drunk that he could barely walk, he slammed my head into the car window, bit my forehead, and then held a gun to my head. I didn't think I would live past that night. I prayed he would pass out, so I would feel safe and because I knew I had to leave.

The next day, I went to work before he woke up, and I left him. I filed a restraining order and for divorce. It was not easy, going through with it, because of the fear I had to live in. He didn't leave me alone for about a year, and I was absolutely terrified of going anywhere by myself. I would shower with the curtain open and turn the water off when I was putting soap on or shaving, so I could hear if he'd somehow gotten inside. Even going into a store would make me nervous. I was constantly looking over my shoulder. I made sure that I was never by myself.

Living like that was miserable. About eighteen months later, I took a leap of faith and moved to Austin, Texas. It was time for a fresh start in a place where I could live without constantly looking over my shoulder. I needed a new beginning.

Fresh Start, Same Wounds

Moving to Austin, Texas sure felt like a fresh start for me. I fell in love with the city, its jogging trails, the hill country, the night life, and the variety of activities that were always going on. It was a whole new world to me, compared with where I came from. I had visited Austin a few times, but living here felt so surreal. I felt really free in Austin.

I was no longer going about my day, looking over my shoulder to see if he was there. For a moment, I almost forgot about all of the pain I had been carrying with me. I even thought I had run away from it for good. If only it worked that way.

I began a new career in real estate and mortgaging, and I had a whole lot to learn. As the newness of living in Austin started to wear off and I began to settle down to truly make a living for myself, I started experiencing some not-so-fun symptoms in my body.

It is naïve to think that our emotional burdens have zero effect on us physically. I was unaware of this fact, though, for far too long. I had to learn this lesson, though, when all of the emotional pain and limiting beliefs began to take a toll on my physical health and well-being. Your physical health is greatly affected by your emotional health. Our bodies digest everything, and then it all must come out in some way. It is up to us to choose a healthy release.

Stress actually weakens your immune system, which makes you more susceptible to getting sick and to autoimmune diseases, all of which I learned the hard way, as you will come to find out.

I was diagnosed with IBS (irritable bowel syndrome) and started having horrible reactions to most foods. Saltine crackers, rice, and oatmeal were about all I could eat. I began suffering from general anxiety disorder. I had zero clue at the time what that was. I felt trapped in my body at this point.

My body was crying out for help, but I just thought it had turned against me.

I began to watch what I ate and exercise regularly, and my symptoms greatly improved. I got into a serious relationship, and for a moment it seemed like everything was going to be okay.

Eighteen months later, I had my first child, my sweet boy, Brady J. I was a mom! I loved every single moment and never missed one second of his life. I never knew I could love so much or feel such an undying, unconditional love. I felt this for the first time ever.

When Brady was two years old, I gave birth to his little sister, my precious sweet girl, Bryndle Lynn. I was twenty-nine years old. Up until this point, after overcoming the anxiety and irritable bowel syndrome, I had felt fine. But when Bryndle was around five months old, I began having horrific panic attacks, along with anxiety around my menstrual cycle every month. There was only one week a month when I felt good. I was diagnosed with PMDD (premenstrual dysphoric disorder), which is a severe case of PMS.

I honestly was so frustrated at my body and thought I was cursed. No one else I knew suffered from any of those horrible symptoms, so no one could relate to what I was feeling. My husband at the time did not understand and made me feel like it was all in my head, which did not help.

I started to feel ashamed for struggling with anxiety and PMDD. No one should ever feel ashamed about struggling with their health and mental symptoms.

I started to learn about supplements and cutting gluten out of my diet. Doing those things made a difference. I exercised routinely, as I always had, and felt I was healthy, according to what I knew at the time. But knowing what I know now, as a nutritionist, I realize I wasn't as healthy as I thought I was.

My body was asking me for help through the symptoms I was experiencing. The stress had become too much. The Universe was trying to give me subtle wake-up calls, but I wasn't picking up the phone. I just tried one Band-Aid after another, while fighting my own body. I was so frustrated with my body. I felt like it kept letting me down. As you can imagine, that toxic way of thinking helped not at all.

People look down upon mental symptoms and diseases. Shame is often attached to them, so many people do not admit they suffer from them. The word "mental" alone makes people take a step back, like something is wrong with you. Honestly, all that does is make the suffering worse.

I had so much emotional sadness and pain built up inside of me that it continued to bleed into every area of my life. I could have anxiety and panic attacks at any given time. I tried all sorts of therapy, but nothing worked. I did not want medication, because I was told by my spouse that medicine for mental symptoms was for weak people. I simply felt stuck.

As a mom of two toddlers, trying to run a household and help run a business, I didn't feel like I had anywhere to turn.

When you describe to someone how you are feeling and what you are going through, what you are really after, for the most part, is simply to be heard. People tend to feel the need to "fix you" or "have a solution," but when they cannot relate, they simply nod and tell you to feel better soon. I have had that experience way too many times.

All that is ever needed when another person is confiding in you, especially about their health, is empathy. We need true empathy, where the listener puts themselves in your shoes and imagines what you must feel like inside, and then sympathizes with you. For all of the "fixers" in the world, please know that handling these situations this way is as close to "fixing the problem" as you can get.

Being told that it is all in your head or that you are bringing it upon yourself is quickly engrained in you. I believed there was something wrong with me, which added more hurt to my unhealed wounds.

I had absolutely no clue that all the bad memories, pain, sadness, and unhealed wounds we stuff deep-down inside turn into poison in our body. Your immune system suffers, along with your gut and your cognitive health. Then, you are living not only with all of the emotional baggage, but also uncomfortable physical health symptoms. Think of it like a waste basket: if it is not emptied then it overflows.

If all of that wasn't enough, my body began reacting to the toxic relationship I was in. Your gut tells you everything; it's the listening part that fails. We think our heart knows best, but our heart reacts based on what wounds need healing. My waste basket was long overdue for emptying, but I just kept putting more trash in until it burst at the seams and went all over the place. I had ignored my body's plea for help for too long.

At what point will you finally have enough? At what point do you stop living in the past? The moment when you become aware of the invisible chains that have been holding you back, along with the limited mindset that has been keeping you from breaking those chains.

It is hard to look at ourselves from the outside looking in. We effortlessly notice other people's downfalls, pointing each of them out as if we are perfect. Stop using other's shortcomings as a crutch to minimize your own issues. It is time to turn your finger away from everyone else's faults and point it at yourself. Facing your own internal chaos is key in order to heal past wounds.

*****

Takeaway: *Pain is like a bullet hole that you try to cover up with a Band-Aid. It is going to keep bleeding in your life until you pull the bullet out and let it heal.*

CHAPTER 5

The First Catalyst of Breaking the Chains

The disease that turned my life upside down and awoke my inner warrior: time to make a choice.

MY BODY FINALLY CALMED down. Having that panic attack, anxiety, and PMDD was really scary. Going gluten free, plus taking vitamins, minerals, and fish oil for the first time ever really seemed to help. It was a breath of fresh air to feel "normal" again. Through hard work, self-discipline, and dedication, I also was able to lose the thirty-five pounds I had gained during my second pregnancy, which was much more stubborn coming off than when Brady was born.

At that moment, I felt better than I ever had. Business was finally starting to go well, I was in tip-top shape, I felt good, and I had two precious, happy, healthy children. Was all of the emotional pain still there? Yes. Staying busy and having two toddlers will distract you from pretty much anything. By the time your day is done, you are wiped out! Repeat the next day.

Little did I know, my days of feeling good were about to come to a halt!

Every time this particular memory comes up, I am reminded of how fragile life is and how, at any given moment, your life can change.

Living as I did in the Texas Hill Country right outside of Austin, we have many deer, and deer ticks are prevalent. I love being outdoors, and connecting with nature has always been my favorite way to center myself and relax. I lived on a multi-acre property with tons of room to play. I also love running, and we had plenty of space to exercise. I could run around my property and squeeze in exercise on busy days. Brady was three years old at the time and Bryndle was one, so I got my running in any way I could.

One morning in April 2012, I woke up with a bullseye rash on my right inner thigh. At the time, I had not heard of Lyme disease, so I ignored the rash. Little did I know I was one of the lucky few to react to a tick bite this way, as only thirty percent of those diagnosed with Lyme first develop the bullseye rash. The rash did not hurt or itch. It faded away over a few weeks, and I never thought about it again.

About a month later, I got a horrible headache, which was not common for me, plus I started to feel super-fatigued every day, even though I was not doing anything different. By September, I also started to have anxiety again, plus brain fog, and the fatigue grew worse. I went to a few hormone doctors who said my adrenals were fatigued and that was the cause of my symptoms. It all made sense, so I took the doctors' recommendations for supplements.

Nothing helped. I had no clue I was suffering from much, much more than adrenal dysfunction. I had breast implants put in in October 2012, and I believe that surgery made my full cup of systemic inflammation overflow. Three weeks later, I could no longer function.

Fast forward to November 2012. Life as I knew it ended.

It was two days before Thanksgiving. I was going to host dinner for the first time ever, which was a big deal for me. My family was coming into town the next day, and I was not prepared. Between my mom duties, work, and feeling awful, I hadn't even made it to the store yet.

So, I went to the neighborhood grocery store two nights before Thanksgiving to get groceries. I'd felt a little off that day, and on my way to the store I started to have an out of body experience along with major anxiety. I knew this grocery store like the back of my hand and have shopped there countless times. However, that night, it felt like I had never been there before, like I was underwater, trying to see what was going on above the surface.

My list. My list of what I needed from the store was all I could try to focus on. My hands were shaking, my heart was racing, and I felt faint. I held onto that list like it was my life raft. I was confused as to where the items were that I needed and freaking out about why I couldn't remember or why I felt so disoriented. *What was happening to my body? This isn't good.*

Inside, I felt like other people at the store somehow knew what was happening to me or that I looked off, because I was so disoriented. Funny how we can think that, somehow, other people know what is going on inside of us or what we are thinking.

It took all I had to finish at the store and get back home. Never had I felt anything like that, and it was scary! I was terrified. Come to find out I was experiencing derealization. Derealization is pretty much what it sounds like. It is basically severe brain fog due to an inflammation of the brain. Severe brain fog can cause confusion, disorientation, short-term memory loss, lack of concentration, and an overall feeling of emotional numbness. All of which I was experiencing and would continue to live with for a few more years. I found out a year later that I was terribly sick with Lyme disease and the bacteria had infected my brain.

I crossed my fingers that a bath and a good night's rest were all I needed to feel normal again. I prayed I would wake up the next morning and all of those horrific symptoms would be gone.

No such luck. In fact, it was worse. On top of which, I was sweaty, had diarrhea, and felt a panic attack once or twice an hour. You can only imagine the sheer terror consuming me, which made anxiety worse.

I told my then husband, but that was no comfort. I felt like I was crazy, and I sounded crazy, describing my derealization. I was very naïve at the time, not knowing that anyone would ever question someone's health. When your own partner and family do, it cuts like a knife. I was told to be calm and that my freaking out was making it worse. Being told that, along with the lack of empathy, made me even more scared of what was happening in my body.

When it comes to your health, fear of the unknown is absolute hell. That became the definitively worst Thanksgiving of my life. Not many of the people who were there registered any concern for me. It was more like, "What is wrong with her?" but not in a good way. I felt my feeling unwell was merely annoying to the others, leaving me to feel very isolated and alone.

The kids and I went back home with my parents for three weeks, while I tried to figure out what was wrong. I could no longer function on my own, and my husband at the time was too busy to work and be a babysitter. In what seemed like the blink of an eye, I went from functioning to non-functioning. Seven months after that initial bullseye rash, life as I knew it ended and my nightmare began.

How could I not function, you might ask? The symptoms of Lyme disease are vast:

- ✓ Severe brain fog that leads to derealization
- ✓ Severe panic attacks
- ✓ Confusion
- ✓ Memory loss
- ✓ Lethargy
- ✓ Body aches
- ✓ Headaches
- ✓ Joint pain
- ✓ Anxiety
- ✓ Heart palpitations

Don't you think my body was screaming at me through those awful symptoms, tell me something was wrong? I was sure a doctor would know what was wrong and fix me, right? Not so much. Over fourteen months, I went to countless doctors and came away with no answers.

I was diagnosed with hypothyroidism, imbalanced hormones, adrenal dysfunction, depression, and anxiety disorder. I was prescribed all the Band-Aids, but nothing helped. I began to hate telling a new doctor that anxiety and depression were a few of the symptoms, because they were quick to offer anti-depressants and anti-anxiety medications. Even those doctors thought I was crazy. One doctor was certain I needed to be put into medically induced menopause, their answer for getting me well. *What*? I was at the ripe old age of thirty-one!

I knew there was something much bigger going on in my body, but no doctor would listen. They all looked at me like I was crazy. I was thirty-one years old and had gone from being a healthy supermom to needing a full-time nanny. I could barely even bathe myself. I was a shell of a woman. The one thing I was so proud of, which was being a great mom, was taken away from me.

Twice I had the standardized conventional test for Lyme, and it was negative both times. Conventional medicine failed me. Tell me, how is one supposed to know that the standardized test for Lyme is crap? *How*?

Lyme disease is called the great imitator, because its symptoms mimic many other diseases. It can affect any organ of the body, including the brain, nervous system, muscles, joints, and heart. In fact, patients with Lyme are frequently misdiagnosed with chronic fatigue syndrome, fibromyalgia, multiple sclerosis, and various psychiatric illnesses.

Thankfully, I found Functional Medicine. Functional Medicine resonated with me, because it looks for the root cause of your illness instead of giving you Band-Aids to deal with it. I wanted to find the root cause because I knew, in the bottom of my heart, it was more than just imbalanced hormones. When the doctor told me that my symptoms sounded like Lyme disease, I said that the testing with conventional medicine was negative. That was when I learned about the different, more accurate testing available.

I tested again. I had Lyme disease, eight different strands. Since it had been in my body for a while, it was labeled chronic Lyme disease, which is even harder to treat. I started researching Lyme, and what did I find? A bullseye rash. I remembered that damn rash from April 2012, the one I'd ignored.

Lyme wasn't all that was going on in my body, I discovered. I also had heavy metal toxicity, anemia, hypothyroidism, adrenal dysfunction, systemic candida, and leaky gut. It was a lot of diagnoses to take in, but there was also relief for me in finally knowing what was making me so damn sick!

The relief I felt quickly vanished, however, when I was told there wasn't an easy way to get rid of Lyme; even knowing which treatment would help was impossible. What a bittersweet moment, to find out why you are so sick and then to find out no one quite knows how to get you well. But at least I finally had confirmation that I wasn't crazy and none of my experiences were just "in my head," although I had been told that many times by "loved ones."

The doctor started me on the standard treatment, which was the antibiotic Doxycycline. After a few months, I was sicker than before. I didn't know at the time, but antibiotics kill the good bacteria in your gut and flare up candida, which causes an overgrowth leading to worsening of symptoms. My doctor also had me working with a nutritionist to learn how to heal my gut and eat according to the results of my food intolerance test.

I tried two other types of treatments, but experienced no improvements. At this point, I was two years into my illness. If you are wondering how on earth I got through this horrific season of my life, it was my inner warrior. I was not aware of it yet, but my inner warrior kept me fighting and searching to get well.

Rock Bottom

I got pregnant unexpectedly, which was a shock to me. I was so very sick, I didn't understand how that could happen. As if I wasn't in enough pain, I lost that baby at eleven weeks. I had to have a DNC done, and I felt like my body was a garbage can again. I was told, after my miscarriage during Lyme, I would never be able to have any more children.

At this point, I had completely forgotten what it felt like to be human. It is so hard to be that sick and to watch everyone around you live their life. I would often look at my loved ones and wonder, "What does it feel like to feel good?" The days were so incredibly long, just a miserable blur. There was no enjoyment for me during this time. I had tried everything, so I thought, but nothing had worked, and my symptoms were getting worse. I could no longer stand living while feeling the way I did.

My two oldest kids were five and three at this point, and the emotional pain I felt not being the mom they deserved was excruciating. I couldn't walk a few blocks in our neighborhood without paying for it for days. I would watch our nanny at the time play with my kids, and all I wished for was that, one day, that would be me again. Day in and day out. Every single second of every single day was pure hell. Not one single minute of reprieve for over two years. Not one.

So, after feeling invisible and not good enough throughout my entire life, I was now dealing with an invisible disease. The isolation, depression, and anxiety from the disease made me not even want to live anymore.

I could no longer carry the weight of the pain caused from the emotional turmoil, physical symptoms, and mental turmoil that Lyme Disease gave me. Day after day, I suffered with little to no emotional support or understanding. My belief in ever feeling normal again was gone, while others could not comprehend how sick I was. There is no real way to describe the hell I endured. But some part of that, I understand: I believe it is incomprehensible.

Imagine life as you know it today being ripped up from under your feet. You feel like you have been put in hell with no way out. I can offer no better description for the pure agony, pain, and mental anguish of living with this wretched disease. All I know is that I never knew a human could ever feel such horrific symptoms or that our bodies could do this to us.

When I tried to tell people what it felt like to have Lyme, the judgment was written all over their face. Well-intentioned friends and family struggled to comprehend the extent of the suffering of my living with an invisible disease, and this led me to even more feelings of loneliness and frustration.

I would force myself to push through pain, fatigue, and discomfort just to participate in everyday activities, work, or social events. I was constantly hiding pain behind a smile. Anyone suffering from an invisible disease puts on a brave face to avoid burdening others or to maintain a sense of dignity. That constant facade takes a toll on our emotional well-being. Just because you can't see someone's symptoms does that mean they don't exist. What no one knew was that, every night when I went to bed, I prayed I wouldn't wake up the next day.

In March 2014, I was driving alone and came upon an overpass. I suddenly panicked, because I couldn't remember where I lived or my kids' names. I had already been suffering from memory loss due to inflammation in my brain, but this was too much.

I'd reached my breaking point. I felt I must also be invisible to God, because He would never allow one of his children to feel the way I felt and live that way. I was angry at my body, angry at everything. I almost veered myself off that overpass, so I could stop the suffering I was certain would never go away.

I finally made it home. I went straight into my bathroom and got on my knees to pray. I prayed, screamed, and cried to God. *Why? What did I ever do to deserve this? Why is there always some sort of struggle for me? Why does everything have to be so fucking difficult? I can't do this anymore God. If you don't take me, then I will end it for myself.*

As I cried and felt like there was absolutely nothing left of me, I remembered my two precious babies. They deserved so much better than me as their mom, as sick as I was from Lyme. I prayed again. I told God there was no way He would have blessed me with those two angels for them to have a mom be so sick.

I had reached my absolute bottom, rock bottom. With my kids at the forefront of my mind, I felt a fight in me that I hadn't felt before. I told God, if I was going through this wretched disease in order to get well and help one other suffering person, then to send me through it.

I was shaking, because I was damn pissed. I was mad at the disease, mad at what it did to me, and I was angry at what it had taken from me. I got up and went to my vanity mirror. I did not like to look at myself at this time, because I didn't even recognize who I was.

I looked in the mirror and said, *"Fuck Lyme, fuck you. You took over the wrong damn body. It's time to get the fuck out!"*

I chose to believe I could get well. I stopped accepting that Lyme was my fate. I stopped giving any attention to the naysayers and anything negative about Lyme.

Pure Determination

There was a mental fight inside of my head every day from that moment on, once I decided I would get well and not give up. To put into perspective what I was dealing with, there was the combination of all the nasty symptoms from the Lyme bacteria, its toxins, the heavy-metal toxicity, hypothyroidism, leaky gut, candida overgrowth, adrenal dysfunction, and hormonal imbalances, any one of which is enough to make someone want to crawl inside a dark hole and never come out.

But in order to not live in that dark hole, I had to constantly fight all of those nasty symptoms in my body and still somehow mentally fight for something I didn't even know existed, which was to get well and beat Lyme disease.

Everything I did know and had proof of was that I was very sick and there was no cure. I didn't have any proof I could ever get well, but I had faith. An unbreakable faith that awoke my inner warrior. I wanted to get well so badly that not one darn thing would stand in my way. I no longer cared what anyone had to say about it. It was my life. *My one life!*

I took my health into my own hands. At this point, I had nothing left to lose. I felt that the bacteria had made it into my body, and I would make a way out for it. There had to be a way to kill it. So, I began researching. I started researching essential oils for treating Lyme disease. I had to read and reread everything multiple times because of my mushy, foggy brain, just so I could retain it. I knew I could not take any more antibiotics to treat Lyme, because they kill off the good bacteria in our gut, plus antibiotics flare up candida, and I didn't want to feel any worse than I already did.

I bought every book I could on essential oils and read every article I could find online. There was something about the oils that felt good in my gut, to my intuition. I learned what to take to break the biofilm that protects the Lyme bacteria, what kills the bacteria, what helps me to detox and stay calm.

I also learned all I could about the lymphatic system. If the oils were working, then lots of nasty bacteria along with all of its nasty toxins would be floating around in my body, and that would not be good for me. This meant I had to make sure my body was constantly able to detox. Your lymphatic system is your body's detoxification system, and it needs your help to move things along, in order for toxins to be released from your body.

My analytical brain has to understand every little thing, which means I dissect everything. There are times when I tell myself there are some things I do not need to understand or give my energy to; other times, my analytical brain serves me well. I have always loved learning about the human body and how everything works. I had forgotten about that until this moment with Lyme disease, when I wouldn't stop researching the ways for me to get well.

Once I felt I had learned all that I could about essential oils, I bought what I needed. Still, it took me over a week to start using them. Honestly, I was a little scared. What if? What if they hurt me? Oh, I was listening to the fear in my head and the fear of others. How about, what if they work? What did I have to lose at this point? I could no longer live in my body, enduring the horrific symptoms for 86,400 seconds every single day without reprieve. People thought I was crazy for putting those oils into my body, but the oils were either going to work or kill me, and I was fine with either.

The shift in my mindset reminded me of what I wanted so badly, which was to get well.

Time to Die

I began taking the essential oils twice a day, every day. I didn't feel anything different in my body for the first two weeks. But then, what happened after two weeks of taking them? I had my first die-off. How did I know? I knew it was a die-off because every symptom I had was magnified ten times. Just like I had learned in my research. My symptoms during this time were off the charts, feeling like pure hell. I was terrified. Plus, there was that lingering fear of whether I was just getting sicker and it was not a die-off...

About a week later, I felt better! It was a die-off! I knew it for sure because nothing had ever made me feel better over those two long years! Thank goodness I saw the die-off through and did not stop, when it began.

Oftentimes, people quit a treatment when they experience a die-off, because their symptoms get worse, so they think they are getting worse, too. The tricky part of a die-off is that your symptoms temporarily get worse when whatever it is making you so sick begins to die.

What would you do if you were that sick and took medicine that made you feel worse? You would stop. And I believe that is why many people do not overcome and get well, because our natural reaction, when we feel worse from taking something, is to *stop*! I knew, if what I was experiencing during my first die-off was just that, then the temporary worsening of my symptoms would stop within five to ten days, followed by an improvement in my symptoms prior to die-off. If it wasn't a die-off, it would not let up.

I continued with my essential oil treatment. Two weeks later, there came another die-off, and then, five days after that, I had more improvements in my symptoms. This cycle continued for over four months.

I was not cured overnight, but I had a fire lit inside of me that did not allow me to give up. My inner warrior was awoken, and I became unstoppable on my path to healing and getting well. In my continued research, I learned a lot about food. You are either feeding disease with the foods you eat or fighting it. That was foreign to me, but at that point, I would have eaten grass to get 100% well.

The oils were just part of getting rid of the Lyme bacteria. I had to do a complete overhaul of what I was eating. Eighty percent of our immune systems are in our gut, so healing my gut was *key*. The nutritionist I had been working with put me on a paleo diet, which meant no dairy, legumes, corn, grains, dyes, or artificial sweeteners. Going from gluten-free to paleo brought me zero changes or improvement for me. Still, I kept constantly researching health, day in and day out, almost obsessed with it, because I wanted my life back!

I started learning about the ketogenic diet, reading every article and book I could. There was story after story about the ketogenic diet helping people who were really sick. I learned that sugar feeds all diseases, regardless of the source of sugar, whether it's from fruit or candy. I was eating a ton of fruit at the time, especially high-sugar fruits.

I decided to starve Lyme out. I said I would not make my body a place for a disease to survive, only for *me*, Janna, to thrive. I began eating a keto diet, which consisted of tons of healthy fats, clean protein, wild-caught fish, dark, leafy greens, tons of veggies, cultured food, and occasionally low-sugar fruits, like berries. I made my own bone broth to help heal my gut, and I took collagen powder, as well.

Finally, I'd found the missing piece of the puzzle. Between the oils, using food as medicine, starving the disease out, and working on my lymphatic system for detoxing, I slowly got well. Some days were still tough, especially when I had die-offs. There were times when I felt really bad for a week straight, and I thought I was going backward in my healing. But I stuck to what I was doing, determined not to give up.

Little by little, I got well. Slow and steady plus being gentle with my body were key. Anytime I pushed myself too far, it would set me back for days or even a week.

I completely eradicated Lyme disease from my body. I could feel it leave. Some experts do not believe it can be fully eradicated from your body, that it merely goes dormant. I chose to believe differently. Thank goodness I did. After Lyme was out of my body, I then healed my gut and my thyroid. I was able to get off of thyroid medication, too.

I asked God to show me a sign: if I was completely healed, to show me by blessing me with another child. He did. I got pregnant in April 2015. Broden was born December 31 and is as healthy as can be.

For the longest time, I wished I had been aware of Lyme disease. Then, I could have avoided the hell I was going through, and my kids would have had their mommy fully functioning for those few years. What I have learned is that this experience was a vital part of the growth and development I needed in order to uncover my purpose.

I cannot express enough the importance of empathy and compassion in supporting individuals with invisible diseases. I encourage you to listen actively, offer assistance without judgment, and believe the experiences of those who may not "look" sick on the outside. I hope for greater awareness and understanding of invisible diseases by shedding light on these conditions and sharing my story of resilience.

JANNA JOHNSON

*****

Takeaway: Lyme disease was almost the death of me. It brought me to the depths of hell. It also brought me to my knees. The day I almost took my own life to end the suffering was the day I said F*CK LYME! I chose to live. I chose to believe I could get well and eradicate Lyme from my body, when everything told me that was not possible! I won, and I left Lyme in the depths of hell, where it took me.

*****

I wrote this poem about Lyme disease about seven years ago. It took many years after I got well for me to talk about my journey with Lyme or even to write about it. I had a fear, after I got well, that if I spoke about it or relived it any way, somehow, I would get sick again.

That fear has only been gone for the last four years. Writing and music have always been very cathartic for me.

*****

My Why

I never thought of food as medicine.
Until I had no choice,
When Lyme ravaged my body
I had to find my voice.

All I wanted to do
Was to find the magic pill,
So that I did not have to suffer,
I no longer wanted to be ill.

Doctor after doctor but still no cure,
I had to find something,
I was dying, I knew for sure.

JANNA JOHNSON

I started to study, read, and listen,
I was not going to give up,
Lyme might have taken over my body,
But it did not take my hope.

I learned sugar feeds all diseases.
So, I cut it out in all forms,
Along with legumes, grains, and dairy
Eating veggies, fat, and protein was my new norm.

The Lyme now had no more ammo.
It started to die away,
It took over the wrong body
I killed it day by day.

The struggle was real,
But you could not see my fight within,
Nobody knew how sick I was
Until my story touched them.

Lyme did not define me,
But as I look back on it now,
Lyme put me on my journey
To help others know how.

To use food as medicine
Puts your health in your control,
I will teach others, that is now my role.

Janna

CHAPTER 6

The Cost of the Victim Mindset

There is no winning with a victim mindset, only staying stuck and powerless. It is in the victor mindset where you can move mountains.

IT WAS HOPELESS. For over two years, when I was so sick and debilitated from Lyme disease, all I wanted was to hear a story of hope from someone who had been as sick as I was and had overcome it. I searched everywhere for that success story, reading every single blog article, comment section, social media private groups for Lyme—you name it. Every single day I couldn't find a story of someone overcoming this wretched disease from hell, I died a little more inside.

I was all alone in my personal hell. You might be thinking surely, I had someone in my life comforting me and motivating me with hope. No, I didn't. The only humans who kept me going were my two precious toddlers, Brady and Bryndle. But they were too young for me to talk to about the disease. I did my best every day for them, pretending I wasn't as sick as I was.

All I had was myself and my faith. At the time, I didn't even know the term *victim mindset*. Some people might be thinking, "Janna! You had Lyme disease! Of course, you had a victim mindset!" I most certainly had a victim mindset for the two years of the disease, but if I had stayed in that mindset, I would not be well today, I know that for a fact.

Look, tough times are certain for all of us. Your first natural response to any sudden hardship or heartbreak is to think, *What just happened and why? I don't understand. This doesn't make sense. Why me? Why is this happening? What did I do?*

Just don't get stuck in that thinking. Let yourself react just as you should, but don't get stuck in your reaction of shock, pain, and grief, because that is when you acquire a victim mentality.

Being stuck in a victim mindset relinquishes your ability to overcome and succeed. You give away all of your power when you succumb to it. In so doing, you create a vicious cycle of unwanted events in your life, which you invite in through your victim mentality. When we "assume" something bad is always going to happen, it does.

As unfortunate events happen, they continue to feed and give control to the victim mindset, which then allows the process to repeat itself. The more this happens, the more defeated and beaten down you feel internally.

Having a victim mindset makes you bitter and hopeless. You eventually lose all faith or hope for positive outcomes, and you expect only negative ones. It becomes a poison in your life and chains you down to an unfulfilled life of misery.

With a victim mindset, the adversities you encounter, which were sent to be your teachers, you turn into tragedies. Do you really want to live that way? Are you that scared of flipping the switch to a mindset where you are the victor?

Always remember that your actions will follow your thoughts. That doesn't mean, if you state a want or desire a few times, it happens. I would love to win the lottery, and in fact I say that a good bit, but I never buy a ticket to even have a chance. All I was doing, by voicing that I would love to win the lottery, was simply make a statement. For over two years with Lyme, I always wanted to get well and even voiced that. Of course, I did. But again, I was just making a statement.

What was missing? What was so different about me wanting to get well versus that pivotal moment when I chose to believe I would get well? *Belief and determination.*

Everyone who suffers from a disease, sickness, setback, or hardship wants to get well and not suffer anymore. That is a given. No one wants to be uncomfortable, but on the other hand, not many people want to feel more uncomfortable in order to not suffer. It is a matter of which discomfort you want. Again, you can want something all darn day, but if you don't believe the outcome, your desire is already there for you. If you are not determined to claim it, then you will never have it.

The moment I chose to believe I would beat Lyme and would not accept anything else set fire to my determination to do so. For over two years, what I was missing was the belief I could get well, until I shifted my mindset and said, "F*ck Lyme! You took over the wrong body, and it is time to get the hell out!"

You have to stop asking, "Why me?" and start asking, "What do I need to do?"

There was nothing easy about the road I took to get well. Make no mistake. I didn't know if I would ever get well or how long it would take. I couldn't see any light in that dark tunnel I was in for a long time. My brain was so infected with the Lyme bacteria, and my depression, anxiety, and brain fog were so severely intense, it felt like I was in a constant battle with demons and had no weapons. What I didn't know was that the biggest weapon of all was my mind, and that was all I needed.

After I got well, I remember reflecting on that moment when I chose differently. I realized, as soon as I made that decision, my actions followed every single day. Our actions follow our thoughts. Never had I thought that my mind had such an impact on what I did.

That was the moment I realized the power of our thoughts. I wasn't the same person I'd been before Lyme. I viewed life so much differently than before. Never doubt one's will and determination. We all have great excuses sometimes to be the victim, but you need to start giving yourself motivation to be the victor. Life can absolutely suck sometimes and throw us curveballs that are shitty.

Having lived with an invisible disease for a few years will toughen you up a bit and give you a different perspective on what truly is important. I look back now, nine years later, and Lyme is just a little part of my life. I am very grateful for it and for all that I learned during that difficult season. Shifting to a victor mindset had the most beautiful prize, and that was me beating Lyme, which then allowed me to heal myself 100% from everything else Lyme did to my body. I got my life back!

There is no prize in a victim's mindset, but there is a cost: your life and the quality of it. You stay stagnant when you have a victim mentality. It is impossible to overcome anything that way. Stop feeling sorry for yourself. Remember that you cannot always control what life throws your way, but you can control your mindset, which is what will lead you to overcome.

In order to avoid getting stuck in a victim mindset and instead to develop a victor mindset, use these powerful tools, which have led me through some tough times:

1. **Grace**: Give yourself a grace period, allowing yourself a day or two to process your feelings and thoughts, anytime adversity comes your way.
2. **Control**: Control only what you can. You cannot control what happened, but you can control how you get through it, which greatly affects the outcome.
3. **Blame**: Do not place blame on anyone or anything, as doing so puts you in a victim mindset.
4. **Focus**: What outcome do you hope for in the situation at hand? Focus your thoughts and energy in that net result you hope for.
5. **Resilience**: Stay strong in your effort and mindset. All you can do is your very best. Know that not every day is a step forward; some might feel like you took ten steps back. Never give in to giving up.
6. **Trust**: Trust in the outcome and in the power of your mindset. Trust in knowing that your life has already been laid out, but it is your belief and mindset that determine the results.

Thank goodness I broke out of my victim mindset. Looking back on when I was so sick that I couldn't function, starting on that night when I was in the grocery store before Thanksgiving, I see I had no clue what was happening to me. If, in that moment, I had been told I was going to have to endure the hell I was feeling for two-plus more years, I would have said there was no way I could. Up until finally receiving my diagnosis, all I dreamed about was knowing what the f*ck was making me so damn sick!

When the diagnosis of Lyme disease came, I had a feeling of relief, but it was quickly shattered when I learned there was no apparent cure. Setback after setback. I was alone, judged, criticized, talked about, made fun of, and not believed.

I was married with two children, almost two and four years old. My partner did not know what to do with me except offer me criticism and questioning, making me feel it was all in my head. My family lived six hours away, and at the time they also questioned me and were confused about what to do. Anyone whom I thought was my friend wanted nothing to do with my new situation.

I had nothing except a shitty disease with no known cure and a shred of faith that was hanging on by a thread. Lyme disease gave me my mental strength. Hell, it gave birth to it. I am thankful for that. It tested me, it brought me to my knees, and it showed me who really cared about me. It taught me food was my medicine or poison, how to heal my gut, all about the lymphatic system and nutrition, that it can be killed and eradicated, and about how much I am capable of overcoming.

Can you learn all of that with a victim mentality? I don't think so. There was no one holding my hand, guiding me on the path to wellness. No one. I grabbed my own hand and carved my own path. Looking back on all this, nine years after I beat Lyme, I am still amazed I made it through that horrific time by myself. But something happens inside of a person when they overcome the greatest odds all alone. I didn't just win the battle against Lyme; I won the war of my mind.

If I can go through that hell and come out on the other side, better than I was before, then so the f*ck can you.

*F*ck Lyme, f*ck disease.*

*****

Takeaway: *If you are ever defeated, let it be because you fought. I will be damned if I go down without giving it my all. We all have our last day, so make sure, on that day, you know you gave it 100% and nothing less.*

CHAPTER 7

Perfectionism is a Mask

Stop spinning your wheels striving to reach what is unobtainable, you will never achieve it. If you want perfectionism, then embrace your imperfections.

STOP SETTING YOURSELF UP FOR FAILURE! Start setting yourself up to win, to achieve, to conquer, to be happy, and to be free of all that is holding you back. When you do that, then you have really set yourself up for life.

Perfectionism is fake and unachievable. Stop wasting your time. The idea of perfectionism will change constantly, based on what society deems as perfect in the present moment. Just as you think you are about to achieve that current idea of perfection, it changes, leaving you chasing after it again and again. How tiring.

We are all guilty of falling into the trap of trying to be flawless and perfect, but at some point, you have to realize it is just a trap. A trap put into place by insecure, narcissistic, wounded individuals who are scared to death to show the raw, real version of themselves. Hell, they probably don't even know what that is, anyway.

So, they hide behind the mask of perfection they have created, in order to shield themselves from anyone ever knowing who they really are. They have hidden from their own selves for so long, they are lost. Anyone who is confident in who they are will terrify those who wear the mask of perfection, and so, they prey on them to make themselves feel better.

This mask of perfection creates puppets who are so desperate for approval, they succumb to doing what is deemed flawless in the present moment, just to be approved of and fit in. Social media feeds this part of our ego with filters in apps, where you can look like anything you want while removing your "imperfections." Fun as these filters can be, they are not reality.

The cold, hard truth is that perfectionism is just a cover-up of internal chaos and pain. It is a way to get others to "look over there and not over here." It has absolutely nothing to do with anything internal, just external. It is like driving by a beautiful house with the perfect, manicured yard, but when you walk inside the house, it is dark, dirty, and in disarray.

Perfectionism is simply a means to deceive others about who you authentically are. But the only person being deceived is yourself. You are deceiving yourself that you can obtain true happiness and life of fulfillment while wearing a mask of perfection.

Being perfect is not achievable. No two people even have the same idea of what perfect is anyway. The media, social media, and the opinions of others are what have contributed to the idea of perfectionism from the outside looking in. That is all fake, and no matter how hard you try to reach that "idea," there is always a new look, item, or thing that is considered perfect in the present.

Instead, start thinking about perfect from a different lens. Start looking at perfection from the lens that you are perfectly imperfect, what works for you doesn't need to work for others, and the goals you set are achievable.

Do what is perfect for you in the present moment that you are in. Stop putting things off because you think you can do it better some other time, because when you do that, you normally end up never doing it. The idea you have for perfectionism is halting you from even trying. For the longest time, if I didn't feel I gave a 100% every single day and to the full extent possible, then I felt I was half-assed that day. That is not a good mentality to have. All that way of thinking did for me was make me feel like I wasn't doing enough or wasn't good enough.

Now, I have adopted a new mindset on what giving a 100% means to me on a daily basis. I now give everything I do and approach every single day based on what I actually have to give that particular day. Some days, maybe all I have to give, physically, mentally, and emotionally, is sixty-five percent, fifty percent, forty percent, or even ten percent. But I give 100% to exactly whatever that level may be. So, if all you have to give today is thirty percent, physically, mentally, and emotionally, then you give 100% of your thirty percent available! Most important is to be perfectly content with that.

It is truly amazing how just shifting our mindset on the way we think and perceive has such a huge impact on how we feel and on our outlook on life. The idea that this was even possible was foreign to me, until a few years ago. What? We can actually control how things affect us and choose what we give our energy and power to?

Be gentle on yourself and give yourself grace, when you don't feel good, when something goes wrong, or if you are having a hard time. Being your own worst enemy and critic is not going to help. Take this advice from someone who still struggles with this herself. I am much better than I used to be, and I will continue to get better, now that I know I am capable of changing anything I want to change.

Outward perfection is typically what people are after. The way we look, what we have, what we do for a living, and how much we make. If it was all internal perfection, then I wouldn't even need to write this book. That was such a huge eye-opener for me, when I realized the definition of perfection that many people are after. It is how we want *others* to perceive us.

But how do *you* want to perceive yourself? If you achieved your idea of perfect, would you be happy? Would you have all that you could ever want? Does it include how you feel inside? Or do you think, once you reach being perfect, you will finally feel happy?

Striving for internal "perfection" is where the gold is. Focus on that, and everything else falls into place. From here on out, perfection means improving and doing the very best you can in the current moment. No more comparing yourself to anyone else. Looking at what everyone else is doing and comparing it to where you are is not beneficial for you. I learned that putting my focus and energy into my life, with blinders on to what others were doing, made me more productive in my life and less critical of myself.

Honor who you are, the way you look, the way you think, the way you feel, and where you are in this very moment. Thank your body for all it has done for you and for all it is doing. How often do you thank your body for all it does for you, each and every day? We criticize ourselves and get mad when our body doesn't feel good, but you also need to be thankful for all your body does for you!

Let's think about that for a minute. We are constantly attracting, whether we know it or not, and if you are in a low vibrational state, then you will attract just that same frequency. You also put yourself in a state of vulnerability, which makes you a target.

A target for what? The predators that sneak into your life and constantly take from you; the only thing they ever give back is disruption. They come in the form of emotional vampires, narcissists, and energy suckers. They sniff you out from a mile away. It is easy to see whether people are confident or insecure. Those predators are no match for a person who exudes true confidence, and they know that.

I know I am too much, too much for the wrong person, and I am just fine with that. It is only when we are insecure with no confidence that we crave everyone liking and accepting us, because each person who likes you gives you a little boost to your ego.

How much weight are you carrying around? A heavy load or a light load? I am not talking about how much you weigh on a scale! I am talking about the weight of shame, unforgiveness, and guilt. Many of you also carry the burdens of others. Living your life, feeling like you are carrying an extra thousand pounds on your shoulders, is not healthy. It is absolutely taxing and stressful. You might not even be aware that you are dealing with that extra stress, but you are. Emotional burdens take a toll on your body.

What is the self-sabotage spiral? It is a relentless effort to punish yourself for what you have deemed punishable. This is typically anything you are ashamed of and carry guilt about. You give yourself consequences for not maintaining your mask of perfection. You self-sabotage, but then, as you continue to do so, you create a spiral that spirals more and more with each punishment.

The spiraling becomes a hungry beast within us that needs more and more to overcompensate for our self-defeating thoughts that poison our minds. You begin to believe every fear, insecurity, and ridicule of others. You become trapped in the prison of self-sabotage, defeating yourself without even giving yourself a chance. Your flaws are all that you are aware of, and you forget your strengths.

The self-sabotage spiral is comparable to a tornado. It gathers from a storm and then continues to pick up strength as it destroys all that is good until there is nothing left to tear down. The longer you allow it in your life, the more it destroys.

Storms are going to come into our lives, it is just the way life is. The key is learning how to weather those storms and get through them with as little damage as possible. Rainbows come after the storm, as soon as the sun comes back out. The same is true for the rainy seasons of our lives. You can numb your way through those tough seasons, avoiding the lesson at hand, or you can learn from it.

Too many of us deal with internal conflict by numbing. We all have a vice or vices to help us cope and not think of pain.

As if our bodies do not have enough to take care of, we pour toxins into it, hoping that toxins will drown out our own toxicity. Have you ever thought about it like that? What is your vice?

- ❖ Overeating
- ❖ Undereating
- ❖ Alcohol
- ❖ Drugs
- ❖ Sex
- ❖ Over-exercising
- ❖ Workaholism
- ❖ Constant social life
- ❖ Social media/technology
- ❖ Constant binge watching
- ❖ Shopping obsessively

These are just a few examples of vices used to numb ourselves. But why? Because it is easier to keep pushing down the things that have hurt us than to face them. We, as humans, want to be comfortable, constantly. We do not want to face the events and memories that hurt us. We just fail to realize that no matter how much we try to push away our pain or try to forget it, we simply cannot outrun it. All the numbing in the world won't make it stop.

More than just trying to numb away your pain, the other reality is that most people have no idea how to "fix it." I believe most people really want to heal all that haunts them, they just don't have the tools to do so.

The idea that pain can be your teacher, and you have the ability to turn it into a positive seems asinine. I get it. You have to deal to heal. Until you deal with all of the negative crap you are holding inside, you might be self-sabotaging to cope. Numbing yourself is not a solution. It isn't easy to face your demons, but it is a necessity if you don't want them anymore.

My Body Became My Garbage Can

In my mid-thirties, I suffered from another eating disorder. Having suffered with anorexia and bulimia in my teens and twenties, I had no clue that the overeating I had begun was an eating disorder as well. I use the term "overeating" because that is exactly what I thought I was doing.

However, I was doing much more than that. I was hiding in the pantry, typically when I was home alone or at night, when everyone was asleep. I would eat gross amounts of anything and everything until I almost vomited. Once I reached the point of vomiting from eating so much so fast, then the feelings of guilt, shame, and embarrassment came over me.

Binge-eating disorder is no joke! People take it lightly and laugh, but it is serious. Most people don't even know what it really is. There is a huge difference in overeating and in binge eating disorders.

I had no idea of it myself or the severity of it. *Binge-eating disorder* (BED) is the number-one eating disorder in the United States, according to the National Eating Disorders Association. It's a common eating disorder among men and women, especially women in their mid-thirties. Most do not realize they even have it, because overeating becomes a way to deal with stress.

Binge eating is when you eat an excessive amount of food in a short time ignoring the amounts until you are so full you feel sick. These are symptoms of BED (binge eating disorder):
- Episodes of compulsive overeating, of feeling guilty for it, and then punishing yourself by not eating for a period of time.
- Obsessing about how you eat, the way you look, and body weight.
- You have at least one binge-eating episode per week for at least three months.

What triggers binge eating is negative thoughts and habits—which is why it is also referred to as *emotional eating*. That is exactly what I thought I was doing in the beginning: emotional eating. I would get so upset with myself and disappointed at my loss of control and for sabotaging my body.

This became a vicious cycle, until I realized that all the food in the world was not going to take away my stress and the emotional pain I was trying to numb. I was most certainly not going to feel as healthy as I wanted. I was going through an immensely stressful time in my life.

So, what gave? I got sick and tired of fighting my own self. Tired of using my body as a garbage can. Eating that way and the feelings afterward just made me feel worse, and I didn't need that.

I was tired of trying to achieve some level of perfection that I had in my mind! Why was I doing that to myself? I realized I was in charge of the expectations I set for myself, so why the hell was I making these unachievable expectations? I felt gross inside my own body, but I was the only one to blame.

I went to my full-length mirror to take a good look at myself, but not the way I normally did. No more shaming myself and picking every flaw apart. What good had that ever done? I realized it was all of the critiquing of myself that had led to one eating disorder after another. I never once looked at myself and liked what I saw.

Never had I approved of my own self! Wow. It sank in real hard, and I cried at how awful I had treated my own body after my body had given me three healthy babies and healed from Lyme disease! That is pretty remarkable, in my opinion, and I never once just appreciated any of it. The thing is, when you truly do treat your body like the temple it is, everything really starts to change. You don't mistreat yourself when you love yourself.

It was time to start appreciating my body. It took a lot of work to start having a healthy relationship with food. I had used food as a reward or consequence my entire life, and that is no way to live.

I had to detach the shame from binge eating. It was really hard for me to have a cheat meal or splurge on food and not feel guilty. There was a lot of healing to do there.

I now can enjoy a splurge meal and not freak out mentally and punish myself for it. It is so very important, especially for us women and young girls, to teach our girls to just love their body exactly the way it is. It is okay to want to improve your body, but you will get to your body goals a whole lot faster if you love yourself and your reason for improvements is a positive one.

Ready to stop self-sabotaging and finally embrace yourself? Start with these steps and be gentle with yourself:

1. Number one is truly just accepting. Accept that this is what it is and where it is right now.
2. As negative thoughts come into your head, acknowledge the thought and say, 'Thank you for reminding me of what I don't want and what I don't need." Then, replace it with a positive one.
3. Stop making unrealistic goals. Start making achievable goals! No one is going to lose twenty or forty pounds in a month. Don't set yourself up for failure.
4. Stop comparing yourself to anyone! None of us are made the same, and we're not meant to be the same.
5. Be happy with what you accomplish at the end of each day. Say thank you to yourself and show gratitude for your accomplishments.

You don't have to set so many goals for yourself. It can just be a daily goal of doing better. For example, today I want to cut out sugar, and tomorrow, I'm going to work out, even if it's just fifteen minutes. If you say, I'm going to start working out an hour every day and you haven't been working out, that's not going to happen. But you can do five or ten minutes every single day. Don't think that's not enough time to work out, because anything is better than nothing!

Remember, when you set achievable goals, they are reachable! It's such a mind game that you end up just giving up altogether. So, if you set unrealistic goals, you're probably going to give up.

*****

Takeaway: *Your imperfections are your gold, your own personal unique footprint, things that only you have.*

CHAPTER 8

The Eye-Opening Final Catalyst

The beautiful thing about being completely broken is that you can put yourself back together differently. A new you can be born!

"NO! NO, NO, NO! This isn't happening. It can't be, not to me! Not to my precious babies. Why the fuck do I constantly have to be hurt? I need a break. I cannot deal with this one, God. Please, take it away! I beg you, please! My heart can't handle this."

I was thirty-eight years old and by myself in my car, heading from Austin to Oklahoma, about a nine-hour drive. I was crying and praying out loud while trying to see the road through my never-ending tears.

I was certain it was just a nightmare, and I would wake up from it any second to the life I had known. But that would never happen, because I wasn't having a nightmare. It was all real. I had just found out the most earth-shattering news in my marriage. I never saw it coming. I had suspected it, but denying it always gave me hope. The confirmation of my suspicion was unbearable. The emotional pain was the worst

I had ever felt. My worst nightmare was coming true. I was in shock that this was actually happening. This was my life.

I felt like I couldn't breathe. The betrayal brought up the feelings I had struggled with my entire existence, *that I wasn't good enough and something was wrong with me*. I couldn't bear feeling like that for one more second in my life! I'd finally had enough!

This time, when that old insecurity reared its ugly head, it wasn't welcome. I said, "Hell, no!" I am enough, and there is nothing wrong with me. The tears poured out, soaking my entire shirt.

It took all those years of getting hurt and worn down for me to realize it wasn't my fault. None of it was. I was guilty of being my own worst enemy, guilty of not loving myself, and guilty of putting up with too much shit. But I would be *damned* if I was ever going to take the blame for anyone else's shit and wrongdoings again. I was at a new level of pissed. I was angry, infuriated, and numb, all at the same time.

I pulled over, since I could no longer see through the tears flooding my eyes and blurring my vision.

It was more than the betrayal in my marriage that created the flood of tears. It was the accumulation of every damn painful memory and experience I had ever had. The tears were spurred of the root cause of my limiting beliefs: insecurities, attempted suicide, eating disorders, and self-destructive bad habits.

I was remembering all those devastating moments I'd never deserved. All the abuse from the first husband, whose painful memories still haunted me. I thought of the hell I'd lived in when I was so sick with Lyme disease and never knew if it was my death sentence or not. The loss of a baby and pain of having a miscarriage. I'd made it through some dark rough times in my life, none of which I deserved, but they'd happened nonetheless. The only thing I could do about any of it at that point was to forgive all of it and move on.

Carrying it around with me like they were open wounds wasn't doing a damn bit of good. They needed to heal. I needed to heal. I never should have put others' guilt on myself in the first place. The reason I carried those burdens was because I thought, if I was good enough, then none of them would ever happen. Why had I done that to myself? I put up with shit I never thought I would and ignored my gut, while being told it was all in my head. Never again.

This is where I learned what forgiveness truly meant. Until this point, I thought forgiveness was for the other person, accepting that what they'd done to you was okay. That is not at all what forgiveness means. Forgiveness is for you, not the other person. Forgiveness has nothing to do with whether what was done to you was okay or not. It means that what that person did is not on you, it's on them. Regardless of the extent of the wrongdoing.

How long do you want to hold onto unforgiveness? Whether you choose five years, fifteen years, or fifty years, that is how many more years you will carry the hurt. The pain won't stop eating you up until you forgive. Until then, all of the hurt will have a negative effect in your life until you do. The realization of this hit me hard. I had carried so much pain around letting it bleed into my life.

The only way to stop carrying around all of those burdens is to forgive who and what caused them and to forgive yourself. I forgave myself and all of it, every fucking thing. Damn, did it feel good to do that. Those burdens were not meant for me to carry in the first place.

How much dead weight rests on your shoulders that shouldn't be there? It is time to forgive and cut the dead weight off you are carrying around.

Fuck This Shit

There is something powerful that takes place when you reach rock fucking bottom. The perfect storm hits you, and something inside of you clicks, causing the light to shine on all the bullshit you have been blinded to. They say love is blind, but I don't think that is true. It is our insecurities, fears, and desires that make us blind to the red flags, which are clearly visible, but we choose to overlook them. The reason we overlook them is because we don't love ourselves enough.

Love is not blind. The lack of love for ourselves makes us blind.

Upon that realization, I knew that, unless I made the necessary changes and healed myself, I would continue to be blind to what was not good for me. The pain I felt was unlike any other. It took my breath away, along with my ability to fall into the old victim mindset. I was flat-out fucking tired of giving in to the lies and excuses. Where had they gotten me, anyway? Settling for bullshit, that's it. The tears that day were different. They were not tears of feeling sorry for myself, but rather cathartic tears. Cleansing tears that showed me there was another path for me in life to follow.

Was it the pain from the ultimate betrayal? Or was it the accumulation of every single heartbreak and all the adversity that opened my eyes to it finally being time for a change? It was all of it for me. Every damn bit of it. I was sick and tired of giving all of me, only to be crushed and discarded. A transformation of me and the way I approached life was long overdue.

It was time to confront my weaknesses, insecurities, and demons. I needed to make myself a priority for once, and learn who the hell I was, not who I thought I needed to be in order to please someone. My inner strength had gotten me through the darkest moments of my life, but now it was time to use my own strength to create the life I wanted and to become whom I was meant to be.

There is something beautiful when you hit rock bottom and are brought to your knees. This is where you can clearly see through all of the bullshit and learn what you are made out of. My biggest teachers were at the bottom in that pit of hell, but it was for me to choose that. The pain can be your teacher or your chains. Reflection was my lens to all that I would no longer allow in my life. My give a f*ck was gone.

For over a decade, I gave all of me to being a devoted wife and mother. I allowed manipulation, put downs, lies, and being torn down to shreds, while still trying to be perfect. For what? Love and acknowledgement. I was always told that I was the problem, something was wrong with me, or I was too much. No matter what, nothing I ever did was enough.

All the dreams and aspirations I voiced were always squashed. I felt dumb every time I voiced one, followed by immediate regret for saying anything. I started to feel that maybe my dreams were stupid. I continued to push down any part of me that was frowned upon, like my honesty and quirkiness.

My self-esteem and self-confidence were gone. For the longest time, I tried to be everything I thought was wanted. I just wanted happiness, no matter the cost. Looking back on that time now, I realize that every part of me that makes me stand out, my footprint, are all the parts that were disliked. No wonder I felt so empty. I could do nothing right. Even the betrayal was somehow my fault. Yes, it was wrong, I was told, but if I had been happier and more laid back, then other things wouldn't have been so tempting. No accountability on their part, whatsoever. To say I felt worthless and used is an understatement.

I got used to being home alone with the kids for the most part. I was well aware what working late entailed. The pain and sadness I felt daily was deep. I might have put up with more than I ever thought I would, and most certainly never will again, but I needed to be able to look at my precious babies and know I'd done all I could. Each time hurt more; each day that passed carried the reminder that the inevitable was near. But with the pain came a numbness that made me no longer give a shit.

Every punch in the gut gave me strength to finally stand up for myself and have self-worth.

It was high time to stop putting up with all of it. It was time to stop believing the lie that things would ever go back to "normal." Besides, I realized that what I considered normal was not fucking okay anymore. I didn't want to go back to how things were. I finally saw that I wasn't happy, wasn't able to just be me, and that my relationship really wasn't healthy.

It's funny how you see things differently when you stop taking the blame for everything. These were all the thoughts swarming around in my head. I cried while reflecting and realized all that I had chosen to turn a blind eye to. I couldn't live like that anymore.

My ex-husband knew my triggers and exactly how to upset me. Probably enjoyed doing it. I was told I was a b*tch for fourteen years, and every single time it made me cry. I would ask why he said that to me, knowing how it hurt. For over eighteen months, I poured myself into therapy, and one of the things I learned was how to no longer allow his hateful words and tactics to hurt me. That was not an easy thing to do.

After being worn down, I finally had had enough of being told that. One day, as I was signing the papers, I told him that once my ink hit that paper, I was done. He said, if he wanted me back, he would. (Yes, this dipshit actually told me, if he changed his mind down the road, he'd get back with me.) To which I quickly responded, "*Never!*"

He then proceeded to say all of the same hurtful things, followed by telling me I was a b*tch. I told myself, "Fuck this shit. I am sick and tired of it."

I wasn't affected by his words that time like I had always been, in the past. I looked at him and said, "You know, you keep calling me a b*tch, and it just occurred to me, we must have different definitions of the word b*tch. So, if your definition is a strong, independent woman who doesn't put up with shit, then yes, I am a b*tch!"

The look on his face was priceless and damn did it feel good for me. He said, "F*ck you!" and left.

There is nothing easy about divorce. It sucks. Especially when kids are involved. For over two years, I had endured betrayal, lies, and heartbreak. I had put on a smile to the outside world, to pretend all was well, but it was fake. I was done pretending in order to appease another person. I was done with being told what was wrong with me and what I needed to change to fit in. I didn't give a shit about fitting in anyway. I wanted to fit in with myself.

Who was I, though? The first time I was at home without my kids, after becoming a single mom, I looked around and realized I didn't really like most of the crap in the house. My opinion never mattered. I had always picked every little thing out to make someone else happy. And I realized, what do I even like? I had no clue, but I was excited to find out! There was a new fire lit inside of me that I had never felt before. I was determined to rebuild my broken self, but not into how I once was. I was going to put the pieces of me together in a new way, an authentic way, and the only way I could truly be me.

Coming out of a toxic marriage was like finally being able to breathe again, after having no idea you were being suffocated. My eyes were wide-open to the reality I had lived in for so long, which had smothered me so much, I'd lost myself and didn't even know who I truly was. It was exciting to rebuild my life and myself; it felt like the possibilities were endless. I felt free, being on my own and being a single mom. I no longer lived under scrutiny and ridicule.

My shattered spirit became strong again, as I carefully and slowly put my heart back together, but this time, it was me who did it. I knew that never again would I *need* someone to fix me: that was my job.

For the first time ever, I felt my own energy. After being told for years that my energy was heavy and negative, this was all I knew. I'd never felt I was that way, but I had never been alone with myself enough to feel it. It felt so damn good to feel my energy. It is light, fun, warm, and loving. My home started to feel like *my* home, with *my* energy, and others, felt it too.

What will it take to open your eyes to change how you live your life? Does a life-changing event need to take place, where your whole world is completely turned upside down, in order to open your eyes? No, but there does need to be a push for change. Something must open your eyes to the desire and need for a new perception of life. If not, then what is going to cause you to want different?

I do believe that the Universe gives us little nudges to change, but when we don't listen, we are pushed a little more. Every little bit of resistance and discomfort brought to us is a push to ignite change. Something must mold you, push you, and prep you for your calling here on Earth. If everything that is meant for you just fell into your lap, you would not know how to handle or appreciate it.

We are given the lessons we each need according to what our purpose is here on Earth. I had to go through what I did to be prepped for my calling. The deciding factor was that *I had to choose* for the lessons to be my teacher! I found myself, and for the first time, I learned to love who I was, my true self. I went through hell and back and still had some rough roads ahead, but I found my wings. I learned that true love and happiness begin in yourself! You must love yourself, accept yourself, and create your own happiness. That is for no one else or anything else to do for you.

*****

Takeaway: *Emotional and mental pain are the catalysts for change. This is the only kind of pain for which there is no medicine, supplement, or procedure to alleviate it. Healing is the only medicine.*

CHAPTER 9

Surrendering: The Beginning of Change

SURRENDERING IS NOT WEAK. It takes a strong, determined mind to completely surrender.

By no means are you giving up; rather, you are giving in to change, growth, and new possibilities. It is in surrendering our need for control, in letting go of our ego's relentless grip on outcomes, that we find a path to serenity and growth.

It takes a lot of resilience and faith to surrender, which is not obtainable for the weak. Surrendering is what allows us to get rid of the heavy load we carry internally that weighs us down and blocks us from what makes us flourish and grow. It is the only way we can open ourselves up to all of the possibilities that are waiting for us. Surrendering offers you peace and allows you to embrace the present.

Close your eyes for a moment, take a slow deep breath, and sit with these questions:

- Am I ready to face all the invisible chains holding me back and break them all, one by one?
- Am I ready to let go of what I think I need, the opinion of others, the outcome I desire, and how I must go about getting it?
- What will I lose if I surrender?

Open your eyes. How does that make you feel? If you were thinking to yourself, "Absolutely not!" then you are not ready to surrender. To surrender does not mean to give in as in "accept less than." It is not something you do every now and then or when convenient. It is a feeling you embody, an inner trust of guidance from the Universe. A strong sense of faith, you could say.

When I fully surrendered, it was like taking a long, deep, cathartic breath. The need for control was gone. Even though nothing about my future or what was to come was certain, I did not feel panic about that. I felt calm with every being of my fiber. I realized how much stress I had put on myself by trying to control every little thing and outcome. I had been focusing on the wrong thing my entire life. Surrendering allowed me to live fully in the present moment and embrace it for all that it was.

For the first time ever, I clearly understood the connection between ourselves and the Universe. I had always believed there was a much higher power in charge, but this was different. I felt a shift of energy and a sense of ease, upon surrendering. It was like the Universe was answering me back.

All of the fears, worry, and insecurities that kept me playing small and holding myself back no longer had a hold on me. I felt so free and light, like the Universe had taken my hand to lead the way. I had a deep understanding of why adversities come our way and that the two choices are to fall victim or to walk through the painful season, allowing it to teach you. When you do that, the Universe answers back, knowing that you fully understand how it works.

In some ways, I feel like surrendering connects us to the Universe with a deep understanding of how it all works. It is like you are finally accepting the invitation that allows doors to open for you, with endless possibilities behind each one.

As I was embracing this new feeling, I was breathing in a feeling that was calm and relaxing, while breathing out all that no longer served me well, it was me saying yes to me, whatever that may be. And if I wasn't guided to what I wanted, then that was okay, because I was trusting that I was being guided to my purpose.

These are the steps in order to surrender:

- ❖ Acceptance
- ❖ Forgiveness
- ❖ Releasing resistance
- ❖ Love yourself
- ❖ Embracing

Why is it so easy for us to surrender to the negative without question? Why do we not question the bullshit, negative crap, and painful seasons? Why do we just believe that all of that is true, deserved, and a life sentence? I am dumbfounded at that thought! We hear or see something trending on social media, and it becomes our new doctrine without even researching the facts. It is time we *start* questioning the bullshit and *stop* questioning the truth.

What we do question is when anything good happens to us. We question the idea of how healing and changing our perspective could change the trajectory of our lives. But it can. I am living proof. Those who question with doubt are not ready. Those who question with hope and readiness are ready. Remember: your actions will follow your thoughts.

Acceptance. Surrendering is impossible without accepting yourself. You must accept yourself for exactly who you are and where you are in this very moment. This is important so you can become who you want to be! If you feel shame, guilt, or even embarrassment, that is okay, too. Surrender *all* of it!

Struggling to accept the parts of you and your past that serve as wounds in your life is like thinking that somehow you can go back and change the past. That is not possible. Acceptance of all of it, the good and the bad, is a necessity because surrender is what makes change possible. Acceptance releases you from the grip of the hurts that have a hold on you.

Forgiveness. This is for you, not for who hurt you. Remember, when you forgive, you get your power back and release it from whoever or whatever caused the pain. Until you forgive, the anger you feel from the hurt stays present, creating stress and suffering in your body. But once you do forgive, the anger dissipates along with the stress and suffering. Do yourself and your body a favor. Forgive.

Releasing resistance. Resistance does not exist in surrendering. Resistance blocks you from receiving what is meant to be yours. It is like being handed a gift and not opening your arms to receive it. Resistance creates resistance. It took me a long time to see that. The more you try to control every situation and outcome, the more you are trying to force the outcome you think you need. Take a second and ask yourself why you desire the outcome you are trying to force. It is time to stop the tug-of-war game with yourself and with all the made-up fears rolling around in your head!

I will be honest with you. It was hard for me to let go of control at first. But every time I started to feel resistance, I reminded myself to let go, without forcing, and to just surrender. Does "fully surrender" mean to let go of control of every aspect of your life? I prefer to be in control of what goes on in my life. I like to be prepared and know what to expect. There is nothing wrong with that, as long as you do not take away your chance of enjoying yourself.

There is nothing more frustrating than being around someone who chooses to not have a good time, or whose mood instantly darkens when a variable pops up in their plans. I have been on both sides of that coin, and I have to say, life is much more enjoyable when you just roll with the punches. Of course, there are circumstances that can arise that truly can put a wrench in the plans, but if it is minor and doesn't change the outcome, then try to be flexible.

Always keep in mind the end result or net goal you are after in any given activity, event, or day at hand. This mindset hack is a great little tool, one of the many ideas I learned, as I went through my own internal transformation.

Divorce is brutal, especially when it is with a person you cannot reason with, so that first year came with a lot of painful moments. At any given time on any given day, something would rear its ugly head that I had to deal with and seemed like a new vampire to my happiness.

Finally, I realized that I could no longer allow those unexpected matters to completely ruin my day. Yes, it sucked, but it sucked more when I allowed it to steal my enjoyment of life. We cannot let every disruption take our joy and peace.

Here are questions to ask yourself that will help you improve your outlook and mood, when a disruption comes your way:

- ❖ Will worrying change anything? (it will only hurt)
- ❖ Will talking about it over and over help?
- ❖ Can you fix the issue right now or even today?
- ❖ What can you do to ensure the end result that you are after?
- ❖ Is the issue at hand really important to the present moment?
- ❖ Is there a work around on the issue?
- ❖ Can the matter you are presented with be put on hold for a day or two?

It is absolutely exhausting to try to control every little thing in your life. Don't be so busy worrying about what everyone in your life is doing that you completely forget to focus on yourself and your own life. There are people who worry so darn much about what is going on in other people's lives, because they somehow think that control will help produce good in their own life. They put forth all this effort into trying to control others because this type of person wants everyone's focus to be anywhere but on them!

One of my wise aunts gave me the best advice one time, she said, "Go by the 3 Cs. If you didn't cause it, you can't change it, and can't control it, then let it go." That is absolutely correct.

Stop giving your energy away for nothing! Meaning, if you give energy to every little thing that bothers you or pops up, then you won't have energy to give where it really counts. Besides, it takes a lot more of your energy to be upset than to be happy. Isn't happiness what we are all after?

Love yourself. No one can fully love you until you love yourself! The reason for this is, when you love yourself, you don't need someone else to do it, so you don't just settle or look for it. The very first thing you need to do, in order for you to take control of your happiness, is to love *you, all of you*! Unapologetically, authentically who you are! All of it. You must embrace your flaws and stop shaming yourself.

You cannot give or teach what you do not embody. So, do for yourself as you would your best friend, child, and loved one. Would you tell them it is impossible to change, that they are not worthy of love, success, and happiness? I hope not! So, why do you want to keep telling yourself those bullshit lies?

What kind of love do you want the most in your life? Do you want unconditional, pure, true love? Because you can only seek out the kind of love that you have for yourself. So, do you love yourself unconditionally? The solution for what you so desperately desire is to give yourself that love you seek.

Embracing. Embracing is the last step in surrendering because now you can *receive*! It is impossible to embrace until you have completed the previous steps. Imagine you are standing with your arms wide-open, ready to receive and embrace all that has been waiting for you! Embracing is the opening of the gate for your path to all of the doors that contain your purpose and desires. Your mind is now open to new ideas and possibilities. You trust the vibes you pick up and no longer force things to happen.

Remember that this is all new to you. You are retraining your brain and how you think, so you will need to remind yourself of this as you go through the process. We are creatures of habit, which means we naturally revert back to what we know, how we respond, and how we do things. Anytime you begin a new habit, you have to stay consistent. It is not any different than working out weak muscles. You have to work out and stay on top of it, in order for your muscles to get strong again.

As I was learning to surrender, there were moments when a new idea came about, and I caught myself naturally shutting down to the new idea. I realized I was reverting back to old thought patterns that were no longer serving me well. I simply said, "No, thank you" to that thought and reminded myself to say *yes*! I had to remember to embrace all the new concepts and possibilities that came my way. Honestly, it was refreshing and exciting to see how it all would unfold.

Feeling calm and light comes when you surrender. We do not realize how much our body holds onto when we carry around emotional pain and negative feelings. Be gentle with yourself during this process. You will crave quiet time with yourself, so allow yourself that space and time. Do not allow distractions to numb yourself and do not give into frustrations.

*****

Takeaway: *Not surrendering while expecting change is comparable to trying to run with crutches. It isn't possible. Surrender so you can receive all that is already yours.*

Chapter 10

Create the Space

You cannot have the new beginning that you are after in the same environment you want out of.

"I AM NOT MAKING any changes until I feel safe," said the person who was not serious about having a new beginning in their life. Call it stubborn, if you will. Or maybe making changes in your environment makes you a little uncomfortable. Either way, the smallest, most subtle changes to your environment and surroundings create a domino effect that causes even more changes, like your thoughts, daily routine, and the choices you make. We are creatures of habit, so the idea that changing anything not internal, like our thoughts are, could really have an impact on us internally seems far-fetched. I get it.

As you begin to work on yourself on the inside, you will begin to make changes to your environment as well. They go hand in hand. Your current environment was created to fit who you were and who you are in the moment. As you get to know your true, authentic self, then you get to discover what you actually like. You will be drawn to what speaks to your soul, and you won't care less if anyone else likes it.

As you begin working on yourself internally and going through this process, reminders are your best friend. What better reminder than changing up your surroundings and environment? Every single day thereafter, you will visibly see changes, which will serve as constant reminders to you to keep going on the journey of healing yourself.

Like that first time alone in my home after the separation, when I realized not only did I not know my own tastes, but I didn't even like the décor and items I had been picking out for over fourteen years! Adjusting and replacing the furnishings and décor in my home served as reminders of who I authentically was and was becoming.

Discovering yourself is bittersweet. It isn't easy letting go of what no longer serves you well, but it is an adventure to discover who you are, what you like, and all of the new experiences!

It is such an eye-opener about the power of the mind! Once you begin seeing and feeling your personal transformation, it all begins to click and make sense. I can compare my thought processes now to before I began shattering my limiting beliefs. Many eye-opening revelations would have been *impossible* for me to even comprehend before!

Never ever settle! I know, without a shadow of doubt, if someone had told me I was settling in life, my stubborn self *never* could have been convinced that was true. And the comment would have ticked me off to no end. Well, funny thing is, it was true. I was settling in every aspect of my life.

Where you settle is where you build your house and live, so make sure where you choose to settle is nothing less than you deserve. You settle because you are scared that where you are and who you are with are as good as it is going to get. Newsflash: there is so much better out there for you.

I couldn't see it then, but it is crystal clear now. What was blinding me was the lack of love and approval of my own self. Until I gave myself that, I looked for fulfillment from everyone and everything, which meant that I settled. I sold myself short, because I so desperately needed love and validation, no matter the source.

Where are you selling yourself short? In relationships, friendships, career, boundaries, or believing in yourself? I was selling myself short in every category.

Let's take relationships, for example. I learned, as I was healing, that it takes a strong person to truly understand me and get me. I tend to bring out insecurities in others, because some people are threatened by those who are 100% authentically themselves. The reason it takes a strong person to be with me and to be a part of my life is because a strong person has also been through some shit, healed from that shit, and grown because of that shit.

Frankly, I need the person by my side who has also grown and elevated themselves by choosing to learn and become a better version of themselves. Why? Because then I know that person will understand me and also help me to get through future tough times, which always come. It is just a part of life. I need people in my life to challenge me, understand me, and give me the room I need to just be me. I will never stop growing and learning, even when I am ninety.

When you are with the right person, they would never let you settle for anything less than you deserve. My friendships are not the same, but that happens when you are no longer the same person. People change, and you either grow together or you grow apart.

Pull the Weeds Out!

In order for you to bloom and have only flowers in your life, you've got to pull the weeds out, babe.

Just like you cannot have a beautiful yard and flower bed full of weeds, you cannot fully blossom and bloom with weeds in your life! The tricky part is, the weeds are sometimes disguised as flowers, like the beautiful flower that stinks to high heaven when it is pulled, because it is really just a weed.

It isn't easy doing this, especially while in a limited mindset. But as you go through this process of shattering limiting beliefs and healing, you will weed out some of those weeds, just because you will no longer be a food source for them. Then, you will not want any more weeds. The hard part can be that one of your closest confidants might not be the flower they present themselves as. I had a few myself. I never would have thought they were weeds, and it was hurtful when the mask came off. As hard as that realization was, I most certainly was glad to know the truth. I outgrew them, plain and simple.

It isn't always easy to see, when you are still in the room, so to speak, but once you are outside that room, you can *clearly* see all of the signs and how those kinds of people work. They attach themselves to a food supply, and you are that supply, until you uncover their truth. Some of my very close friendships abruptly and unexpectedly ended, when I began to change. It was painful and broke my heart. It took a year to heal from that, but I realized those were not my people. The people who are truly for you will be there for you without fail. Never fight for anyone who is okay losing you. Let them go. They don't deserve you anyway.

If you are super-dependent on any figure in your life, then please pay close attention to that. There is a good chance both of you are each other's food supply. That was another realization I had, once I found myself and was healed and finally loved myself. This is because you probably balance out the insecurities of that person you are dependent on, and vice versa; you do not trigger each other. However, once one of you does the healing, you no longer have the insecurities that threaten the person you were so dependent on. They are still dependent on you, but you no longer need them, which can make them feel even more insecure. It is very common for those people to then turn on you, as their way of getting back at you for hurting them by healing yourself! That doesn't sound like a true friend, does it?

Which one is more important to you, *quality* or *quantity*? If you or someone you know cares more about how many friends they have or how many followers they have, that is a big red flag indicating they're someone who needs to heal and get rid of their insecurities. When *quality* is more important to you than *quantity*, it shows, because those people typically have a small circle of super-close friends. While they may have a lot of friends or acquaintances, they keep them at arm's length.

The value of quality will supersede the miniscule amount of value you get from quantity any damn day. I would rather have a handful of trusted close friends than a hundred friends who really do not know or value me.

Remember when I said our environment is a reflection of our self-worth? This is a part of that!

So how exactly do you pull the weeds out?

- ❖ Setting boundaries
- ❖ Knowing your self-worth
- ❖ Loving and accepting yourself. *Remember: this begins exactly where you are right now, not for who you want to become!*
- ❖ Only have so many seats at your table; be sure every single person must earn their seat, regardless of who they are!
- ❖ Shattering your limiting beliefs and mindset to heal yourself and your insecurities. That alone makes the weeds pluck themselves out! *Goodbye!*

Get Rid of Unneeded Pressure

Stop allowing other people to apply pressure on you! What happens when there is too much pressure in something? It *pops*! You are no different, my friend. Needy, nosy, whiny individuals are what I call *pressure-pushers*. They push and push applying pressure, until they get their way.

I know for a fact that the right people, who truly unconditionally love you, never put pressure *on* you. Rather, they take pressure *off* of you! I don't care if that person tells you they love you and just want what is best for you. Your true people would never make you feel guilty for anything, because they do not need something from you to make themselves feel better. This is a fact.

Not everyone should have access to you. Your time and energy are valuable and only need to be used where it is fruitful for you. I have three categories I put people in, based on what kind of access they have to me: open door, screen door, and closed-door access. This tool is very helpful in protecting your peace and boundaries. Let's go over each of them.

Open door. This type of access to you is pretty self-explanatory. These are your best friends, confidants, ride or dies; the ones closest to you, who never question you, judge you, disrespect you, or break your trust. They have an open door with you, meaning they get the full view of your life and all that is going on.

Screen door. My grandma had a screen door, and it was rare that her front door was closed. Both her front and back doors had a screen door, as well. She loved the screen door, because she could see and hear the outside better, smell nature, and catch the breeze. But if she needed to close the main front door that blocked all of that out, to protect herself, she could. All that being said, screen-door access is given to those who haven't earned your trust and are pressure pushers, the nosy, needy people. More people will fit into this category versus all the others.

We all have these in our lives, people we know who are nice, but we might not ever form a close relationship with them. This can also be a family member. People use the fact that they are family as a tool to apply pressure and guilty feelings, because they are kin, which gives them a free pass into your life.

No one gets a free pass. Use this category for those who never do anything that merits the closed door or an open door. Set boundaries by showing what you allow and disallow, staying consistent, without wavering or giving in to their needy demands. They will naturally comply. Be ready for the guilt trip, but just know, it is their own voids and insecurities they are reacting to, not yours.

These types typically love to flaunt your accomplishments to their inner circle for their own boasting and confidence-boosting. Since they seem so harmless, you tend to cater to their demands, because they can be annoying, and you know it is the only way to appease them. Let's get this straight!

Closed door. You know what this kind of access to you is. None. You can visualize this door as a tall, thick, steel door with a padlock and security system, if you want, but no peephole. There is zero access to anyone who gets put into this category. This one is for anyone who has shown their true colors, betrayed you, or hurt you or a loved one. Forgive them first, and then throw away the lock and key.

When I began implementing these categories in my life it made it really easy to not be taken advantage of. The old me would give in, try to appease everyone, and let people stay in my life who should have had a closed door. If there is *anyone* in your life whom you need to use the word *appease* for, then *a-ppease* (please) get them the *fuck* out. I had to do this in my own life. The fake people find the exit door, and the rest begin to understand your boundaries and slowly comply by respecting them.

Boundaries

Boundaries are a must in your life. Boundaries protect you from weeds and predators. They serve like a fence does for your yard. You put a fence around the part of the yard where you want to keep the weeds and unwanted things out. Your backyard is your sanctuary and your family's protected space.

Boundaries protect your inner peace, energy, and time. Having them does not mean you are rigid or set in your ways. It also doesn't mean you are stuck in your ways for fear of change. They are simply tools to what you are willing to accept, expect, give, and do in regards to others and yourself. You don't shut people out, unless your boundaries are not respected. Your limits won't be tested when you make it clear what is not acceptable for you.

Enforcing your boundaries, if tested, only reaffirms that you are serious and they must be respected. The weeds in your life are clear to see and will pull themselves out. Do not give your time and energy when it is not reciprocated. Protect your time and energy, so it is available for what gives back to you. The takers in life will go away, making room for like-minded people to fill your life.

Never feel guilty about turning down invites or requests. Start putting yourself first and protecting your inner peace. Only you can do that. The right people in your life will never make you feel guilty for doing so and will always understand.

You will attract like-minded individuals who also have boundaries. Anyone who doesn't obtain them cannot understand why you have them. On the flip side, you will not want anyone in your life who lacks boundaries. Boundaries help maintain your freedom and prevent your being chained to obligations that you really have no desire to fulfill.

It doesn't make you selfish to have boundaries in your life. Switch that way of thinking about them. Instead, think of it as being selfish *not* to have them, because it is the selfish people in your life who will expect you always to give in to their needs, while not giving a shit about yours.If you do not set boundaries or they are not respected, then what happens is your "inner cup" drains faster and never gets filled back up. I am a huge giver! I over-give to those I love in any way I can. But I had to apply this boundary to my life a few years back, because I was giving and giving until I had nothing left to give, while not receiving anything in return. So, not only were the people I was giving my everything to not returning the favor, but they had mentally and emotionally drained me to the point where I could not even fill up my own darn cup! Do not let this happen to you. Set boundaries.

To clarify, I am not talking about financial or material things, when I speak of giving and not receiving. I am talking about love, respect, appreciation, gratitude, honesty, and loyalty; about someone being there for you when you need them and vice versa. I was always there, no matter what. If I got a call and was needed, I was there. If I was needed to step in and help in any way, I was there! But where were they, when I needed the same thing? I would wait and wait for my calls and texts to be returned, but it was a matter of convenience for them.

I have allowed people to just absolutely run all over me, even walk out of my life without a word and straight-up ignore me. Then, I would forgive and let them back in. What always hurt the most was I knew without a doubt I had done absolutely nothing to merit their actions. I would be terribly confused, assuming it was once again my fault, wondering what was wrong with me, when I hadn't done one darn thing wrong.

I do not have the ability to treat anyone that way, so it was very painful when they treated me like that. The last time that happened, it was by someone whom I *never* would have expected it from. That was the moment when I realized it would *never* happen again. I knew then, no matter how painful it might be, I would never allow someone to walk back into my life, if they chose to walk out.

Here is the deal: Anyone with a limited mindset and beliefs is not capable of understanding boundaries, much less having them. Why? Because, in that shattered mindset, you rely on others to fill your voids, regardless of the disrespect you receive or do to yourself. That is precisely why this topic is toward the end of the book, because you must be, at this point in the journey, ready to set boundaries to protect yourself as you develop strategies to heal your wounds and shatter your limiting beliefs.

It isn't easy to stick to your boundaries, at first. You might feel resistance when you encounter enforcing them the first few time. But you shouldn't, if you are truly committed and determined to the transformation.

If you want to see who truly loves and respects you, set boundaries, and it will be obvious. Boundaries are a form of self-respect and show others what you expect. I decided a few years back that those people who are meant to be in my life would be there, and effortlessly. If someone doesn't appreciate you enough and or realize what they have in you, then don't wait for them to walk out the door. Hell, open the door for them, show them the way out, and then change the damn lock! You do not have a revolving door. Everyone has to earn a seat at your table.

*****

Takeaway: *You need to take control of your life, but to do so, you must take control away from others who try to control you! The Universe will not give you all the abundance in store for you while there are people in your life who will take it from you. It's time to plant new seeds.*

CHAPTER 11

Rejection

When you seek the approval of others, rejection has the power to break you. However, when you only seek approval from yourself, rejection is a welcomed landmark on your journey.

REJECTION FEELS LIKE a punch in the gut. It serves as a reminder to why you have the fears and insecurities you have, reminding you as to why you are lacking. Being rejected reminds you, loud and clear, that you are not enough and never will be, so you might as well give up. *In fact, don't even try! Just stop hoping that, this time, it will work out. It has to— you know did your best.* That little glimmer of hope quickly fades the very second rejection happens to you.

That little glimmer of hope is now gone, and you have succumbed to self-defeat, over and over. Why should you believe any differently? You have all the proof you need. You damn sure don't want to feel crushed again, so not expecting anything good and not even trying are what protect you from rejection. You stick with what you know works and what won't hurt you.

But what happens with that limited mindset of rejection? Protecting yourself is your reason for not pushing the envelope and going after your dreams, but that is your excuse. But what if you change *how you perceive* rejection? With an open mind, putting your limiting belief aside, choose to view rejection as your teacher. Painful as it may feel, it is much more painful to get stuck pursuing something that is not for you.

The sting of the pain might slowly go away, but let it remind you that being rejected is merely a guide on the path to your destination. It serves not as a roadblock but as a signpost, pointing us in the direction of our true purpose.

Rejection is one of our biggest fears. Why is that? No one wants to feel rejected. No one wants to lose, no one wants to feel like they are not good enough, and no one wants to be the one who wasn't chosen. I myself have suffered rejection, but not anymore. I changed the way I think about rejection and making that mindset shift has helped tremendously.

Rejection is primarily a fear of those who have yet to accept and approve of themselves. As long as you seek both acceptance and approval from any source other than yourself, you are allowing rejection to hurt you. The negative context of rejection goes away with acceptance. I know that might sound easy, but it really is, if you just put your energy toward loving and accepting yourself! Did you know:

- ❖ You will never *not* make a mistake.
- ❖ You will never be good enough for the wrong person.

- ❖ You will fail one time or many times before you succeed, but that is how you learn what does not work!
- ❖ You will not be chosen where you are not meant to be.

Rejection is always going to be a part of life, so learning how to overcome it is imperative. You must learn from past experiences, build resilience, and continue to pursue your goals and dreams, despite whatever setbacks come along. Always have a positive mindset, stay persistent, and maintain your self-belief.

Everyone faces rejection at some point in their lives, and it does not define one's worth or potential for success. Do you really want to give any power to rejection when it is from someone who is clearly showing you where you stand in their priorities? Yes, it sucks when you are rejected for a raise, promotion, or acceptance into a program, but you cannot allow any more of your energy to go to that. You were told no for a reason, and you must trust that, as hard as it may be.

So how do you overcome rejection and shift your mindset on what it means to you? The very first thing you must do is validate your own darn self and stop looking for validation from anywhere else. Don't you think you are worth it? I do!

Next, start viewing rejection as simply a landmark on a map to your destination. Whether you grew up having to use an actual paper map on road trips or not, we all know what a landmark is. It identifies a specific place on a map that is easy to see and recognize. It helps you to know where you are, how close you are to your destination, and if you are going the right way.

While it isn't easy to be rejected, especially if it is something you have worked really hard for and thought it was for-sure working out, there is a reason you are being steered away and guided to something different. Trust it, and remember that what didn't work out is for your higher good. It is just a redirection on your path to your destination.

The only rejection you need in your life is to reject bullshit and dipshits.

Time to Listen to a New Tape

I was born in 1981, back when we had cassette tapes that we stuck into our cassette player to listen to music and jam out. If we wanted to record our favorite songs, then we would have our blank cassette ready on a Saturday morning, ready to hit record as we listened to the countdown from our favorite DJ. Sounds old, huh? Nothing better than a mixed tape!

It took a lot of patience, being super-quiet, and a fair amount of time to make a good mixed tape. You were proud of one of those, after making it. But no matter how much I loved my mixed tapes, there would always be new music and new favorite songs. Sometimes, the mixed tape just got worn out and had to be replaced.

Most people have a negative tape on repeat in their head until they replace their thoughts with positive ones. This is another by-product of the limiting beliefs formed in childhood and growing up. That inner critic is tearing you down every single day.

Are you tired of the negative tape playing in your head? It's time to replace your worn-out mixed tape. It's time to break free from the cycle of self-doubt and negative self-talk. Let's silence that inner critic once and for all.

You're not defined by your past, even by your own mistakes or failures. It's time to let go of those negative thoughts and start embracing self-love and positivity. Start loving yourself and being supportive of yourself, just like you would your best friend and loved ones. That inner critic is not your friend. In fact, it is causing you to hold yourself back in life and defeat your own self every damn day!

The good news is that you have the power to change the narrative. How? Becoming aware is the first step. Awareness allows you to start noticing the negative self-talk that's been keeping you stagnant. Challenge those negative thoughts, and replace them with positive affirmations. Remind yourself that you are capable of amazing things. The sooner you start believing that, the better.

Your environment plays a huge role in this, so make sure you surround yourself with positive influences. Surround yourself with supportive friends who truly believe in you and uplift your spirits on a bad day. If your support system looks more like complainers and negative people who feed off of one another, then it is time to reevaluate that circle of friends.

Practice self-compassion. Treat yourself with kindness and understanding. Remember that making mistakes is a part of life, and it's how you grow and learn. Embrace gratitude. Focus on the things you are thankful for in your life, and watch how it transforms your perspective.

You are worthy of love, success, and happiness. Break free from the chains of negative self-talk. It's time to rewrite the script and create a more positive, empowering reality. Start silencing your inner critic, and start giving a voice to your inner cheerleader.

As I was changing out my own negative tape, I would either redirect the thought or replace it. Redirection is when you do not allow the negative thought to stay. You say, "No, thank you," and then redirect to something else. Replacing the toxic lie with a positive truth really helps retrain your brain to a new, positive narrative.

One of the lies I used to tell myself was, "I will never be good enough." I replaced it with the truth, "I am more than good enough and fully capable." Easier said than done, but it doesn't take too long before the new tape takes root and the old toxic one leaves. Consistency is *key*!

Writing down words of affirmation and motivational phrases was helpful for me, and I still write these today. I love using sticky notes. I place them in the bathroom, nightstand, office, fridge, inside my laptop, and anywhere else I can think of.

Every time you see those beautiful reminders, say them out loud or to yourself. Before you know it, you will have created a new tape that fuels your actions. I also write down on these a to-do item that is of utmost importance for the next day as a reminder. Some days, we wake up and just don't feel that great, or the day just doesn't have a good start. Reading my words of affirmation and motivation always helps me to make the most of my day and stay positive.

If you feel silly doing any of this, that is okay! It is new and might seem weird to you. It was weird to me, but I realize now what made it weird was how I was so uncomfortable saying nice things about myself. I had no confidence at all in the new narrative I was creating, at first, but that changed, and it will for you, too!

Every single day, at least once a day, I want you to express gratitude. I personally do this upon waking and at bedtime. You can write this down or simply say it to yourself. No matter how hard my day has been or what painful season I go through, there is always something to be grateful for every single day.

Don't overthink this; there is no right or wrong. Sometimes, mine is as simple as being grateful for my health, the air I breathe, my kids, my husband, my family, the roof over my head, the food in the house, and the clothes on my back. Simple. Showing gratitude is not bragging.

Desires Meet Action

It takes more than surrendering, manifesting, and shifting your mindset for your dreams to come true. However, once you have done those things, your thoughts will make the next step a lot easier. Taking action! When desires meet the right mindset with action, then you can walk through the doors you have unlocked by saying yes to you.

Desires are simply dreams of what we yearn for, deep down inside. Desires give us hope for what could be, inspiring us to a possibility of more. However, without you ever putting action toward your desires, they will remain just that.

The magic is when desires and action meet up. When we take that first step, we began walking toward the door of our desires. Action is what turns your dreams into your reality.

Without action, desires remain only hopes, dreams, and thoughts, and they will slowly begin to fade away over time. If you want to actually experience your life through living those dreams, you must do something about them.

Action is the key that unlocks change, the tool that allows growth and self-discovery. It is a sign to the Universe that you are serious about all that you desire and that you are worth it.

Your desires are the door to your purpose in life, and taking action is the key to you reaching your destination. Instead of fearing action and assuming rejection, view action as an adventure on the path to your dreams.

Every person has desires but that is not enough to make them happen. Simply stating what they are just leaves you standing on the path to the door that has them. But when you take action, you can start moving down the path to the doors waiting for you.

It is easy to say that and easy for me to write it, but I will never forget the day I made the decision to take action.

I was sitting outside by myself, in my favorite spot where I go to think, meditate, and pray. It had been about twenty months since the divorce was finalized. I was reflecting on all that I had been through, all the changes and transformations my kids and I had gone through, and the healing. I was in awe at what can happen in such a short amount of time.

I was proud of myself for shattering my limiting beliefs and for all I had been through in life. I reflected on sitting in that same spot a year before, and another year before that one. What a difference. There was a time when I was terrified at how my life might be in a year, especially while I was going through that painful divorce. What a difference a year makes.

I shifted my focus to think about where I wanted to be twelve months from that moment.

I was ready to embark on a new journey. I loved being a nutritionist and teaching others how to feel their very best, but there was also another calling that had been nagging at me for a while. It had been just a dream. I really wanted all of it to happen, but I was lacking a key component to really go after it. I had never believed in myself.

Something felt different that day, as I sat there, reflecting on everything. There was something I had never felt before: belief in myself. All of the tears, discomfort, pain, heartbreak, triumph, and every adversity I had overcome had prepared me for my destiny. This was the moment. I knew it. I had been questioning the purpose I'd been feeling in my gut, wondering how the hell it was ever going to happen, when I didn't even know where to start or what to do.

That is when I said to myself, "The only person who is going to make my dreams come true is me!" That was a huge moment for me. Never in my life had I spoken that way or felt that way.

I was excited and scared. I had zero clue what to do next. There were negative, self-defeating thoughts coming to my head left and right. I ignored them. I knew those thoughts were lies, lies that had kept me scared to do anything for myself for forty years. I already knew the result of listening to that toxic crap, but I was ready to know the result of listening to the new narrative I had been learning and listening to for a few years, the ones filled with the truth.

I was ready to go after my big scary dreams, which I felt were calling to me. In August 2022, I sat my kids down and asked them what they thought about me going after my *big* dreams. I was a single mom, and my kids had been through enough changes, so it was important to me to hear their opinions.

I think it is important to include our kids in our big decisions, when we can. So much of their lives had been uprooted that I didn't want them to feel like that again. I knew, if I made the decision to go after my dreams, it would take a lot of my time, and I would be much busier when I did have my kids. We had already had to go from being together all of the time to spending only half of the time together, after the divorce.

I shared my soul callings with my three kids:

- ❖ Start a podcast, where I could share my story, teach, motivate, and inspire.
- ❖ Become an author, so I could write the book I had always looked for, when I was sick with Lyme, so others knew they, too, could overcome.
- ❖ Be a keynote speaker, to continue to motivate and inspire others that their mindset is their key to unlocking their success.

I was a little hesitant after telling them that. I had never really voiced it before. My kids' faces lit up, and they all agreed I definitely should do all of those things, should go after my dreams, and that I would be amazing at helping so many people! Their belief and excitement fueled me and will continue to for eternity. In some way, by asking them, I was declaring what I was going to do, because I never would put anything out there verbally to my kids and then not follow through. I would be held accountable!

I had no f*cking clue what to do next. I did not have one single contact in the industry I wanted to be in or even know someone who could give me advice. I knew all of that, but it didn't stop me. I just knew that a whole lot of people do figure it out and make shit happen, so I could, too.

The Universe has a really funny way of letting you know you are on the right path and it is listening. Within one week, I was scrolling on social media and saw that one of my favorite people I follow and had always looked up to was taking applicants for a mastermind of successful, like-minded women who had a story to share and wanted to share it on a stage, writing a book, starting a podcast, or all of the above.

I didn't even hesitate to click and fill out the application. As I was filling it out and answering the questions, I almost changed my mind and discarded it. I didn't feel I had any of those qualities or any of the right answers. I thought there was no way in hell she would look at my application and want me in her mastermind.

I stared at my screen for a while until I remembered the promise that I had made myself. I had promised to no longer succumb to fear and, even if I was scared to do something, I was going to go after it anyway.

F*ck it. I completed it and submitted it. I mean, it wasn't like I was going to get picked anyway.

I was shocked when I got the email from her that she wanted to talk to me over the phone. *What?* During the phone conversation, she personally invited me to join her mastermind. I was ecstatic! I couldn't believe my ears. There was an in-person meeting three weeks after that. I was nervous. I was going to meet her and a bunch of successful women I did not know. I was completely out of my comfort zone.

The event was about a three-hour drive for me. The day I was leaving to drive up was nerve-racking. I was so close to backing out, but thankfully I didn't. That Friday morning, we were all meeting in a conference room at the hotel where I was staying.

My nerves were shot. I was sick to my stomach, and every single fear I could have had was flooding my thoughts. I got off the elevator, and as I turned down the hall to the event room, all I could hear were women talking and laughing. It sounded like a lot of them had met previously and knew or knew of one another.

I stopped dead in my tracks and turned around. What was I doing? I knew no one. I was no one. I was beyond uncomfortable, and all I could tell myself was that, at my age, I did not have to stay uncomfortable when I could choose not to be.

I stood there, struggling not to leave. I was fighting all of the fears in my head, which I had thought were gone for good. But that was the thing. I could fight them, if I so chose to, or I could give in to them, like I used to.

I was too fucking worried about the "what ifs!" *That's right:*

- *What if I don't make it?*
- *What will others think?*
- *What if I am just wasting my time?*
- *What if I make a fool of myself?*
- *What if I am not successful?*

- *What if I fail?*

And then… I flipped the script. I remembered who the f*ck I was. What if I break out of that fucking safety box and my comfort zone.

- *What if I fly…?*
- *What if I succeed?*
- *What if I make it?*
- *What if I change the world?*
- *What if I help save someone else?*
- *What if I show my kids that dreams come true and so can theirs?*

I took a deep breath, turned back around, and entered the room that was waiting for me. I walked toward my dreams and my purpose that day. They were there waiting for me, but I had to choose to go after them, choose to take action, and choose to be uncomfortable. To think I almost walked away and gave into the fears and lies. That was the last day I have ever given fears my energy.

Walking into that room was one of the best decisions I have ever made. It changed my life. I met some of the most amazing women who had also overcome so much and had amazing stories. Lifelong friendships were made that weekend. To be surrounded by like-minded women who just get it is a breath of fresh air. That was the first time I didn't feel judged by women, not one. We all love, support, and respect one another.

I announced to my mentor that my goal over the next twelve months was to start my own podcast. Then, after that,

I wanted to write a book and eventually get into speaking. Five and a half months later, my podcast, *Revive with Janna*, aired. Within that same week, I got a book deal and now you are reading it. Two weeks after both of those milestones, I spoke on a big stage and shared my story of overcoming Lyme disease.

I am not even close to being done. There is so much more I want to accomplish. What makes me so happy is that I did it on my own and by myself, with no direction.

It has been about eighteen months since I walked into the room I almost ran away from. So much has happened in my life in such a short time, after how close I was to walking away, because the fears almost made me believe it wasn't possible. It could have gone either way.

How close have you been to your dreams without even knowing it?

*****

Takeaway*: Stop rejecting yourself. Take any other rejection as simply guides on your journey. Take a leap of faith, and take a chance on yourself. Step into the unknown for new beginnings.*

CHAPTER 12

Taming Your Inner Beast

You can shatter all the limiting beliefs you want, but we all have an inner beast to tame.

"OH MY GOSH, just listen to you, screaming and crying like that. You are crazy? Something is not right with you. No wonder."

Those were the exact words I heard any time I showed any emotion other than happiness or a fake smile. It was okay for this individual to say something hurtful, but it was not okay for me to react. To think I'd had it wrong my whole life!

I am clearly being sarcastic, but that truly was the norm for me. I am no longer in that type of relationship, and you can bet your ass I never will be again. Thankfully, I am no longer purposely enticed to get upset. But of course, I have bad days and get mad at things—I am human! I had to learn that it is okay to be upset and have a bad day and that there was nothing wrong with me.

How many of you do not feel like it is okay to just get pissed sometimes, cry, or scream?

Deep within our souls lies an untamed beast—a storm of emotions that are both calm and fierce. Holding onto these emotions will only cause them to grow bigger and bigger, which will lead to your releasing them in an unhealthy way. In doing so, there will also be unhealthy consequences.

Emotions are not meant to stay trapped inside of you and ignored. Learning how to handle them allows you to stay in control of your emotions, instead of your emotions being in control of you. When your emotions have control, they wreak havoc on you, emotionally, mentally, and physically.

There is power in our emotions, even anger and sadness. Tapping into that power can be the fuel to you taking action and getting control of your life. Allow what you feel to serve as reminders of what you do and do not want in your life.

Taming your inner beast means acknowledging all that you feel and allowing yourself to feel. You must feel and deal in order to heal. It is important to understand how you respond to the world around you. The key is finding healthy outlets to let your emotions out.

By taming your inner beast and not holding emotions in, you free yourself from being tied down and suppressed by emotions. You are no longer scared to feel uncomfortable emotions, and you are confident about overcoming them. This allows you to be more empathetic and compassionate to others.

When you embrace your emotions, you release the fear that accompanies them. Emotions are a constant in our lives, never going away, and we never know when we are going to feel a certain way. So, why not learn how to move and groove with them, so we are never controlled by them?

Anger and sadness are the emotions that make us the most uncomfortable; no one really wants to feel them. So, knowing how to deal with them is key.

Always acknowledge how you feel. I find saying it out loud or writing it down in a journal when I am sad or angry is helpful. Just as long as you take a moment and recognize how you feel.

If your anger or sadness is toward a person then walk away and give yourself space, especially if it is a heated argument or situation. Give yourself a "cool-off" break. Doing this ensures you will not say something hurtful that you may later regret.

Happiness is not a constant emotion. Happiness is just knowing that, no matter what you are feeling today, no matter what you are going through today, it's going to be okay. It's not permanent, and you're going to get through this. But you have to have the right tools in your little invisible mental toolbox, so to speak.

One of the tools we need to have handy is the ability to get rid of that anger, frustration, and madness we sometimes feel. That is what I call *taming the beast*, because you never want to keep stuffing down inside any of those emotions that are not comfortable to deal with.

Every single one of us has had painful, sad, heartbreaking experiences on many different levels. No one's experience is the same. When we go through a painful time, we all compartmentalize the situation. Our brains break it down, so to speak, to help us navigate through the pain.

Going back to the victim mindset again, it is perfectly normal, when crappy things happen to us, to think, "Why on

Earth is this happening?" So long as you do not get stuck in the victim mentality. Please know, there is absolutely no part of this book that suggests you should *never* feel:

- ❖ Angry
- ❖ Frustrated
- ❖ Sad
- ❖ Overwhelmed

If anything, I want you to feel all of the emotions as they come up in your life. What we bury inside of us eventually rears its ugly head. Too many of us do not feel enough! You are stuck on autopilot in *Groundhog Day,* just numbing away!

No more numbing! The key is to find *healthy* ways to let your emotions out. As you find the root cause to your limiting beliefs, go through the healing process, and begin to make the necessary changes, you are going to experience a rollercoaster of emotions at times. Not to mention, life throws us curve balls, so we need to have the right tools to deal and heal. This is *key!*

Most of us deal with our emotions based upon how they were handled in our home, growing up. Maybe you had a parent who yelled a lot, didn't show happiness, took it out on you, or my favorite type, swept things under the rug! You know the type I am talking about. The person who doesn't deal with any disagreement or wrongdoing, the excuse master and reality avoider. My point is, we only know what we were taught, which also means our kids only know what we show them. If we want our kids to be able to express themselves and deal with their feelings, then we must show them how by doing it ourselves!

I titled this chapter "Taming Your Inner Beast," because whatever feelings and emotions we stuff down, put away, and ignore turn into a poison that seeps out into every part of our lives. Those undealt-with feelings become a beast of burden that then is in charge of your life, because until you deal with them, they control you.

I had to learn this the hard way myself, but you don't have to. Crying does not mean you are weak, and screaming by yourself does not mean you are crazy.

While I am discussing this point, let me make one more. If there is anyone in your life who does not allow you the freedom and space to express your emotions without demeaning you for it, then please show them the way out! That is not okay. There are people in this world who are threatened by others' ability to show their feelings. Those are very insecure people who have a *lot* of healing to do. They are toxic and will only hold you back from evolving.

Never ignore what you feel and what emotions present themselves. There is nothing to be ashamed of, if you feel sad or frustrated. I have days when, for no obvious reason, I just feel frustrated. I have learned that, on those days, I am typically putting way too much on my plate. I can overwhelm myself at times, and when I do not meet the unrealistically high expectations that I've given myself that week, I then feel it as frustration.

I have learned to ask myself, why am I feeling what I feel right now? My wonderful, patient, loving husband receives all the credit for helping me learn this. I was super-frustrated one day at all the things I had left to do and not much time left to do it. He gently pointed out that I was being too hard on myself and had put an unachievable amount on my plate.

He was right. Not only can I express myself with him, but he soothes me and helps me. One of the many, many reasons I love him so very much! He is my calm in the storm and voice of reason.

I cannot express enough the utmost importance to have people in your life, especially those closest to you, who truly love you unconditionally and are there for you no matter what. I could not have had someone like him without first loving myself and creating my own happiness. You cannot attract what you do not have.

We all want to feel seen, heard, loved, accepted, and understood, so we must first give all of that to ourselves. How do you want those closest to you to treat you, when you are in an emotional state, whether anger, sadness, or frustration? Think about that for a moment. Have you given that same care and concern to those around you?

We show others how to treat us by how we treat them. Again, we cannot give what we do not give ourselves. So, let me share some things I do to overcome the tough days and the not-so-pleasant emotions that are part of life. Some are reminders, and others are actionable.

Mark this page, make a copy, or write them down, so you have some more tools in your bag!

You have to feel to heal! Next time you feel overwhelmed and run over, try the following:

- ❖ Give yourself grace. It's okay!
- ❖ Give yourself a time period to feel the way you feel. I give myself twenty-four hours to be mad, frustrated,

or sad. I don't always need twenty-four hours, but the point is I do not allow myself to get stuck in a victim mindset. Shit happens!

- ❖ If you need to scream to let out anger or frustration, scream! I go somewhere alone, away from everyone, whether in my car, bathroom, or closet, and I give myself a few good screams. I always feel better after.
- ❖ Get out in nature, if you can. Sit, walk, run, whatever. There is something so healing and comforting about being outside.
- ❖ Write down your thoughts and feelings. Do this in a journal or on a piece of paper. Throw it away afterward, if you want. That is just another way to get it out of you!
- ❖ Talk to someone if you feel like it, but make sure it is a safe space without judgment. I personally like to vent sometimes, but I do not want feedback at that moment. Sometimes, people want to help you feel better so badly, they give advice when you just want an ear to listen.
- ❖ Take a few deep breaths and remember it will pass.

These are the tools I use when I am having a shitty day or something shitty happens, and they help so much! If it happens on a day when I have my three precious kiddos, I typically give myself a few moments, and then I immediately spend time with them, because their love fills me up and reminds me of what is truly important.

I also tell my kids that I am having one of those crappy days and need them to make me laugh! I make sure they know that Mommy has bad days, too!

High Expectations

High expectations of you by others are simply an external tool for fulfilling their own insecurities.

"I expect you to...!"

You expect *what*? This phrase alone makes me think of a person standing before you, pointing their finger in an accusatory way. Who in your life has expectations of you? The first names that come to mind, write them down.

Let me guess: your spouse, your coworker, your friends, your family. What do they expect? Have they voiced their expectations? Or are these assumptions? Are you allowing them to put expectations on you? I wonder how those people would react if you set boundaries?

Keep that thought in mind as we go deeper into high expectations. Let us go back to the burning need for approval and acceptance. That burning need stems from insecurities people have that they try to tame, putting a certain level of expectation on themselves and others. So, take a moment, and reflect on that.

You see, *we put expectations on ourselves that we believe are necessary, in order to achieve the approval and acceptance we seek.* Another way of saying that is to make sure any expectations you put on yourself are not so that you fulfill someone else's.

Let's discuss *others'* expectations of you. If anyone, and I mean anyone, in your life has any expectations of you other than to truly be your beautiful self, they are using that control to avoid their own wounds bleeding on them. They would rather bleed on you. You might need to reevaluate your inner circle. There is a difference between people expecting something from you and people just knowing you and knowing what they get, because they know who you are. People who expect something are typically those people who do not give anything.

Not only did I once have people in my life who expected this and that from me, I also put high expectations on myself aka *high-achiever-itis!* However, the *expectations* I hung over my own head were merely in place to seek approval from others or to tame an insecurity. Now, the expectations I have of myself are simply to always be 100% unapologetically, authentically *me!*

Do not confuse high expectations with having high standards! High expectations are unachievable goals of perfection that are destined for failure, whether they are for you or those around you!

Offended? Disagree? That is okay, because your mindset determines your outlook on that. I would have been offended, hearing that statement in my unhealed, insecure mind years ago.

High expectations are an invisible chain weighing you down. They result from that need of perfection in yourself and in others. Sure, they can be a tool that pushes us to achieve at our highest level, but they typically take a toll on us, too, as we strive for a certain level of achievement.

The toll of high expectations creates unnecessary self-doubt that what you are trying to achieve remains out of reach. This creates unnecessary pressure in your life, which you just don't need, and will wear you down.

High expectations seem like worthy goals, but they are actually a mask of perfection that will hold you back from all that is truly achievable. Remember that perfection is not real and always stays out of your reach, leaving you spinning your wheels.

High expectations will leave you feeling let down left and right, because no one is perfect, including yourself. Once you have shattered limiting beliefs, healed, and broken the invisible chains, your environment reflects all of that, because healing would not have been possible in a toxic environment!

My point is that you then only rely on yourself for happiness, love, and fulfillment, which is reflected in those you allow in your life and how you live your life, so there is absolutely no need or desire for high expectations from anyone! I expect for me to do a little better tomorrow than I did today, or at least to try, and I am not always perfect. Do not put so much pressure on yourself that you explode! All you can ever give and do is the very best you have in that moment.

Stop setting yourself up for failure, and stop setting such high expectations of others that they feel like nothing they do is good enough for you. Set yourself up for success. Make the expectations you have of yourself achievable and doable but not a marker of your self-worth. To be honest the only expectations I had for myself, until just a few years ago, were those that others had of me. We can never stop people from having expectations of us, but we get to decide whether we put those on ourselves. Once you set boundaries in place and the weeds are all pulled out, there should not be many people in your life who "expect" something of you.

I have very simple ones for myself: To always do the best I can with what my ability is on any given day, and to never stop growing and learning.

We all have expectations of how things should be and turn out. But when those expectations don't happen, we are left feeling down and disappointed. As you learn surrender, you will be able to start letting go the idea that everything has to be perfect.

The reality is that we're not always going to succeed, and we are going to make mistakes. Your self-worth is not measured by what you achieve. Your self-worth is measured by who you are as a person and by how you treat others.

Life doesn't always go as planned. In fact, sometimes it goes better than planned, especially when we learn to let go of how we think everything should be and begin to embrace where we are in the moment. So, let's break free from the chains of our own expectations.

*****

Takeaway: *Allow yourself the space and opportunity to feel all of your feelings. All that you suppress eventually comes out, but you only get the chance to choose how the first time. If you avoid it, then your body chooses how.*

Chapter 13

Parenting: With or Without Chains

You have two choices. Shatter your limiting beliefs and heal your wounds or pass them down for your kids to live with them.

"THAT IS HOW I WAS raised, and I turned out fine."

Have you heard that phrase before? It makes me roll my eyes. What I really hear is an excuse as to why nothing should change.

Every single generation should be parenting differently and better than the one before it. If each generation breaks their invisible chains instead of passing them down and also parents their kids based upon how life is during their kids' generation, we will have a society free of so much pain and with a lot fewer problems.

How badly do you want to be a parent without chains? How badly do you want to raise your kids from a healed version of you, instead of the unhealed version?

Whether you are a parent right now or not, this chapter section will open your eyes to how limited beliefs, wounds, and insecurities will continue to have a domino effect on your life and for your kids, until you do something about it.

I was one of those people who didn't know if I would have kids. I didn't necessarily see myself with kids. I will never forget the moment when I felt another life inside of me and knew how right that felt. I knew my first, Brady, was a boy when I was ten-weeks pregnant. I vividly remember thinking about how I was going to parent and what I would do differently, based on things I wished I'd had growing up, plus the things I wanted to pass down, the routines and traditions that I so dearly loved, growing up.

Our unhealed wounds will be passed down to our children, which is not fair. My parents raised me and parented based on how they were raised, mixed with their own ideas, the same as I felt, when I first got pregnant. We all have the choice to change, learn, grow, and do things differently. I always knew, if I became a parent, there were a few things I was definitely going to do differently than how I was raised. Shattering all of those limiting beliefs and mindset was the absolute best gift I could have ever given myself and kids.

I do not want my kids to carry that burden of passed-down, unhealed wounds from me. I cannot protect my kids from everything, but I can give them less to deal with by not passing down my own limiting beliefs. They will have their own experiences and adversities to go through. I cannot stop the storms from coming into my kids' lives, no matter how badly I want to, but I can show them how to overcome and shatter any limiting beliefs that might take root from all I cannot protect them from.

My kids have seen me transform into who I am today. I have hopefully shown them that the uncomfortable times in life are our teachers, if we choose, in order for them to grow and become who they are meant to be. I have absolutely no idea what it is like, as a kid, to have your parents' divorce and find the life you have always known be completely uprooted. That experience alone has planted roots of limiting beliefs and wounds for them. There is no way any human would not be affected by such a life-changing, painful experience. You would be a blind fool to believe any differently.

We have to make sure to let our kids know it is okay to be sad or mad. Their feelings are valid, and they need to feel them. Create a safe space for them to feel what they feel and to share, if they want to. Never, ever make your child talk about something they are not ready to talk about! When you do that, you will scare your kid: not only into telling you, but also that what they feel will get them into trouble. No kid wants to make their parents upset or disappoint them. I make sure they know it isn't their fault! I do everything I can in my power to help ease the pain or sadness they are feeling, but I know I can't make it go away.

One of the absolute worst things a parent can do, when their kid is hurting, mad, or sad, is to tell them they shouldn't feel that way; that it's not that bad, that they are messing up the day. Never say, "Don't be a crybaby," or tell them they are too grown to feel what they feel. Whether your kid is three or seven, eleven or 15, everything they feel is real for them, and they just need you to comfort them. Our kids have to deal with enough crap as it is, in this world they live in, so they most certainly do not need to feel stupid, unheard, invisible, or not good enough in their own damn home and with their parents!

Listen to your kids and validate what they say and how they feel. Every human wants to feel heard and validated. God gave us two ears and one mouth for a reason! Listening is more important and meaningful than talking.

As a parent, remember that you do not know everything, and your experience growing up was in a much different time and age than our kids' today. Yes, there are similarities in just growing up and maturing, but honestly, I think our kids have more hindrances today than we did, growing up. Be open to the idea that you can learn from your kids! Nothing makes my kids feel more empowered and confident than when they have taught me something. Their faces light up like a Christmas tree. They are just little humans whom God entrusted us with to raise to the best of our ability.

Kids are little sponges, soaking up every little detail of life. Let's try really hard to give them as many helpful tools as possible. You should always be growing and learning. The moment you think you know it all is the moment you stop learning.

Our kids can teach us so much, if we let them. My kids keep me young, motivated, inspired, fulfilled, energetic, and curious. I try to give them the same. Parents are teachers, so make sure you are teaching your kids and raising them in a way, so they have the mental and emotional strength needed to be successful in all they do. Having a strong mental outlook and emotional state is more important than physical strength. Anyone can become strong physically, but it is when you are strong mentally and in your heart that you become unstoppable.

Kids are not their parents' trophy, nor were they put on Earth to live their parents' dreams. Do not put limitations on what your kids are capable of and can become. That isn't your job. It is not the job of the parent to direct their kids or tell their kids what they need to do with their life. It is their life!

Don't be the parent who applies so much pressure to their kid to be in a certain profession or be someone they are not. You will make them feel not good enough or that their dreams are stupid. Never, ever make a child feel embarrassed for how God made them and for what He put them on this Earth to do.

We have to remember that, one day, our kids will be grown-ups and able to live on their own. If you push them away and create an environment at home that makes them feel uncomfortable, invisible, or criticized, they will be counting the days until they are on their own. I guarantee it, because that is exactly what I did! I learned from my own growing up and the wounds I had to heal that one of the best things I could give my kids was a safe space.

Their home should be their safe space and their sanctuary. Show them it is okay to have a bad day, to be goofy, sloppy, loud, obnoxious, or whatever it is they are feeling. Home should always be a no-judgment zone. If you provide all of that for your kids, then it is so easy for them to see the difference between a healthy environment and an unhealthy one. We must teach our kids what is healthy and unhealthy in every area of life. If all they know are different levels of toxicity, then they will just choose which toxicity is more comfortable.

I cannot control every part of my kids' lives, especially since half of the time now they are with their father, but I can control the environment I provide for them. My kids know they can tell me anything without judgment and I will never press them for details they are not ready to share.

One of the best things I ever did for my kids and my relationship with them was to let my guard down. Being a parent does not mean you put on a mask of perfection with a whistle around your neck. You do not have to cry or be upset by yourself in the bathroom, so they never see you upset. That is not realistic. But more importantly, how the hell can we teach our kids that not only is it okay to feel those emotions but also how to handle them?

I remember the day I broke down that wall, no longer hiding that sometimes Mommy gets sad and frustrated. My kids showed up for me! They gave me their affection, tissues, and words of affirmation. It was the exact medicine for my soul that day. I realized the importance of showing my kids that I am also human. I also realized that it made them feel good to be able to make their mom feel good.

Empathy is one of the best emotions a human can have and give. We have to teach our kids empathy, so we need to show them. You can never tell somehow that how they feel is invalid. How someone else feels does not have to be valid for you, only for them! It is the same for kids as it is for adults. Empathy does not discriminate based on whether someone thinks their emotions are invalid. Empathy does not need agreement or understanding; it is just simply given.

Kids are going to mess up and make mistakes. They all do. It is part of growing up. Making a mistake is how you can learn. We need to get rid of the idea that, as a parent, you need to come down hard on your kids when they make a mistake. Sometimes, feeling guilt, disappointment, and embarrassment is enough. You do not always have to add to what they feel by interrogating them in a way that brings shame. Never tell your kids you are ashamed of them. You cannot take your words back, so you better make sure you are okay chewing them.

Relatability is the way to reach your kids when they mess up, not criticizing. *Relatability is reachable!* It is the same with everyone, kid or adult. We were all kids once and made some dumb decisions, so let's not pretend otherwise.

Give your precious babies grace and understanding, and then you can reach them in order to teach them! Be approachable to your kids, and they will be sociable with you!

Having kids to raise is the biggest blessing of all. I am beyond grateful for Brady, Bryndle, and Broden. They are my angels and my everything. I promise I will always be there for them, no matter what. I will love them unconditionally and be their biggest supporter and fan!

Make sure your kids know that. They deserve nothing but happiness, love, and freedom. We only get one chance to raise them, and it sure the fuck goes by fast.

*****

Takeaway: When the fire comes, you don't have to walk through it. You can stay in the seat facing it OR walk through it and let it burn the parts of you that are holding you back, so you can be who you are meant *to be. Just remember that the fires you choose to not walk through, you leave burning for your kids.*

CHAPTER 14

Time to Choose

As long as your fears and insecurities are making decisions for you, your life will pass you by. Stop living your life for everyone else, and start living it for yourself.

DO YOURSELF A FAVOR, and stop assuming. An assumption has no facts, it is just what you think will happen. But at this point in the book, it is clear that our thoughts are not always right. When we have a negative tape playing in our heads, then our "assumptions" are based on our fears and insecurities.

As long as I felt I wasn't good enough, I never chose myself based on my assumption. I have always been good enough, and now that I know that, I invest in myself, because I believe in myself. It is time for you to do the same. Stop assuming, start choosing. Stop accepting mediocrity, and start choosing you!

Mediocrity simply means the comfort of fitting in and being just like everyone else. That is boring! Have higher standards for yourself, and strive to stick out from the crowd. If more of us did that, more people would be inspired to do the same. This book is a guide to help you break free from the chains of mediocrity and embrace your true, authentic self.

The path of least resistance is to be mediocre, where you are safe in the shadows of being like everyone else. Stop accepting average just because it is easy to obtain. There is no fulfillment in living an average life. The comfort of an average life will also have regret, unfulfilled dreams, and a yearning that we could have done more with our life.

Choosing yourself is not selfish. It means you recognize your worth, potential, and uniqueness. It shows you are not going to settle for mediocrity or allow external factors to direct where your life goes. It is time to believe in yourself and choose yourself. I know you have the courage to do so. When you choose yourself, you also allow for:

1. Self-Discovery: When you are on the same path as others, you cannot discover who you are. But when you choose your own path, then you are able to discover your hidden potential.
2. Empowerment: Choosing yourself empowers you to take control of your path that leads to your purpose. You take the pen back, so you can be the author of your story. You no longer live to appease others' expectations, just your own.
3. Self-Fulfillment: You only rely on yourself to fulfill your goals, which are for yourself and nobody else. This brings a huge sense of accomplishment as you achieve your goals.
4. Uniqueness: Choosing yourself allows you to find what makes you unique and not fall victim to mediocrity. Staying true to who you are and to your uniqueness keeps your mind open to untapped possibilities.

We worry so much about failing that we don't even try. If we shift the way we think about failure to we don't want to fail ourselves by not trying, then we all would live more fulfilled happy lives. Stop thinking of failure as a permanent outcome. Instead, start viewing failure as a teacher that shows you what doesn't work, so you don't waste your time continuing to do something a certain way that won't be successful or satisfying. Choosing yourself means embracing failure as a valuable learning experience, not as a reason to give up. It's about taking risks, learning from your mistakes, and continuing to strive for greatness.

The saying, "from the outside looking in" is a funny thing. You look at a couple's relationship, and you can clearly see red flags and moral differences. They argue and are just not happy together. You think to yourself, surely, they know those things. Why would anyone put up with that and live miserable?

Well, now I know. It isn't so easy for the person in the relationships to see all the red flags the same way. Remember when I said it is not that love is blind, it is the *lack of love* for ourselves that makes us blind? That's why.

After my divorce and the healing, I then could see things so much clearer, from the outside looking in. Now, I will reject mediocrity in all relationships. Choosing yourself extends to your relationships, as well. It means surrounding yourself with people who lift you up, respect your boundaries, and encourage your growth. You deserve meaningful connections that inspire you to become the best version of yourself. Remember: the weeds will pluck themselves out.

Fuck mediocrity. It is time for you to choose yourself. The rewards are well worth it. Dare to be your imperfectly perfect authentic self. When you do that, you unlock your full potential and live a life that is truly fulfilling. Break the invisible chain of mediocrity, and embrace all that you are. Your future self will thank you, and you will not regret doing so.

Stop Accepting and Start Choosing

Throughout life, we are constantly confronted with a vast array of choices, ideas, and influences. It's easy to get caught up in what is deemed popular by society or what is expected per the definition of others. We succumb to peer pressure and the constant demands of the outside world. But if we quiet all of those external whispers and pressures, and if we start to choose for ourselves, then we will be able to uncover the life we are meant to live, not the one others want us to live.

To blindly accept everything that comes our way and not question it all is to give our power away and give up on ourselves. That is comparable to giving someone else the pen to write our story and choose for us, while we just read the story they wrote.

But when we choose to think for ourselves, we hold the pen and write our own story. We then hold the power to uncover our purpose here on Earth. It's an acknowledgement that *we* dictate our lives, not external forces.

It takes courage to think for yourself. It requires you to question the norm and what the status quo is. However, in doing so, you must pave your own path, even in the face of opposition. This is imperative for personal growth and self-discovery, sending us on a journey where we uncover our true authentic selves, strengths, and purpose.

When we choose and think for ourselves, we build confidence, resilience, and self-awareness. We become better authors of our own story, strictly driven by our passions and desires. It is empowering when we deliberately choose to think for ourselves and live life on our own terms.

So, stop choosing to be content with accepting everything that life presents. Start embracing the power of choice and independent thought.

Did you know you have the superpower of choosing what you tell yourself, what you believe, and what you elect to accept? Choosing is an absolute *superpower*! This might sound cheesy, but there is so much *power* in choosing! You cannot live both ways. You either accept mediocrity or start choosing to overcome and level up.

You would not be reading this book if you didn't want more for yourself. You chose a motivational, inspirational, self-help book for a reason.

I will tell you why. You can read all the self-help, motivational, mindset books and pour yourself into therapy at the same time, and *none* of that will make a difference, because your reason is not in alignment with your purpose. Your reason is not in alignment with learning the lesson at hand and elevating yourself.

Ask yourself this: Are you going to therapy, counseling, and reading all the self-help stuff you can get your hands on because you are trying to fix you? Because there is something wrong with you? That is the reason and motive for most people, and it's exactly why most never truly improve and live the life they are destined to live.

Free will is real. The game-changer is when you choose to grow, evolve, and overcome. It is time to change stuck, stubborn ways that are clearly not serving you well. If you think something is wrong with you, that is the problem. That is a limiting belief. You need to figure out its root cause and heal!

Stop Attaching Your Happiness

When you and only you are in charge of your own happiness, you will never let yourself down! What does that mean anyway, to *attach your happiness*? It means you attach your happiness to people, things, or ideas, giving external factors power over your happiness.

If you do not have those external factors, you are not happy. But if you create your own happiness from within, then you have true happiness, and external factors cannot affect it. Curious if you might be doing this?

Read these statements. Have you ever said any of these before?

- ✓ I will be happy when I get that job.
- ✓ I will be happy when I make more money.
- ✓ I will be happy when I lose weight.
- ✓ I will be happy when I am in a relationship or get married.
- ✓ I will be happy when I have a bigger, nicer home.
- ✓ I will be happy when…

When *what*? When will you be happy? You will be happy, truly happy, when you create your own happiness! You, and only you, are responsible for your happiness, my friend. When you realize that, it's a game changer!

There are so many times when I wish I would have started saying yes to me a long time ago. I looked for self-verification from other people instead of myself. You know, it's like people think, when I have this or when this person loves me or when I get married, I'll be happy. But that's just not how happiness works. You will be happy when you love yourself and create your own happiness.

I often looked at someone or something else for my happiness, and guess what? I was never happy. When you attach your happiness to a relationship, that relationship can't be its best. You can't be your best, because it's a constant drain on the relationship. You're always needing and depending upon your partner to make you happy. That gets really tiring after a while. It's just a vicious cycle, and it constantly repeats itself.

If you are wondering what is wrong with attaching your happiness and your reasoning is, who wouldn't be happier with bigger, nicer things or to be in a relationship? I will tell you exactly what is wrong with it. You are *not* in charge of your happiness when you are attaching it to *anything* other than yourself! You are kicking your own happiness down the road.

If you achieve one of your, "When I...," then you will want or need something else to make you happy again, because the "When I..." is a short-lived, temporary fill for a void that cannot be filled. Once again, you kick your happiness down the road.

If, within one or two years, all of your "When I haves..." come true, you still will not be happy, because the problem is you are not happy with yourself. The "When I haves" are temporary and short-lived. You will continue to look for superficial things to fill a void that needs a beating heart just to love itself.

As a parent, I want my kids to be happy, truly happy! Happiness has to be taught and shown. We have to teach our kids how to be happy with themselves and not to rely on their happiness from anyone else! Especially in this time, when we are all part of an instant gratification society.

A lot of unfair things happen in life, but it's our mindset that gets us through and teaches us what we need to learn. I used to think, once I made a certain amount of money, I would just always be happy. Problems would always be solved, and I could get through anything, as long as I had money.

Not only was that wrong, but I deprived myself of years of happiness, because I attached it, and to something that took a while to achieve! Never again! Instead, what I have learned is that true happiness comes from within. When you are responsible for your own happiness, you don't let yourself down.

The way you attach yourself to happiness plays a huge role in your overall well-being. While external factors can certainly contribute to your happiness, they should not be your sole sources of joy. By creating inner fulfillment, finding meaning, and creating your own happiness, you will lead a more content and satisfying life. So, stop searching for happiness everywhere else except within yourself. The journey of you no longer attaching your happiness is not easy and is always evolving, but it is deep and gratifying.

It's time to tell yourself to be happy, right here, right where you are, and with what you have, with who you are, and with what you look like. To fully embrace yourself. The first step in creating your own happiness is to love yourself. Stop thinking you need more or better. You deserve so much more than that superficial crap. You will find that you need a whole lot less, when you are fulfilled from the inside out!

In the constant hype of life and the outside world, it is easy to get caught up in seeking happiness from external sources. But then, you are attaching your joy to circumstances you cannot predict or control. You can control yourself, though, and how you respond to things. As you create your own happiness within, you will realize you don't even need some of those outside factors.

So, grab the reins of your happiness, and detach it from all external factors—be it material items, relationships, or achievements. You and only you should hold the key to your happiness, not the ever-changing circumstances of external factors.

You will uncover so much about yourself as you choose this. You will realize how you really feel about ideas and life, when you are no longer steered by the pressure of the outside world. You get to choose how you really want to come across to others, and you will find your authentic self.

It is an act of self-love and empowerment, when you create happiness from within. It is an acknowledgement that your inner world is your sanctuary and you do not need others' approval or understanding of your choices. I cannot describe the sense of empowerment and independence I felt when I created my own. I knew that no one could take it from me and that, no matter what happened or what road life took me on, my happiness was intact.

Inner happiness is constant, not fleeting. It is a flame to your inner strength, and it lights your path in life. It resides deep in your soul, solely relying on you and nothing else as its source. It can withstand the tests of time, giving you a source of strength in times of challenge. It remains a source of resilience that cannot be taken.

So, remember, while everything around you will have constant change, your ability to create your own happiness from within is constant and ever giving. You are showing that you choose to live a life filled with positivity, gratitude, love, and self-fulfillment by your own means. When you choose this, you are also showing others the power of creating their own, inspiring them to do so, themselves.

*****

Takeaway: You are solely responsible for what you allow and disallow in your life! Stop feeling sorry for yourself and start fighting for yourself. Stop worrying about hurting other people's feelings and what they will say. Those who are meant to be in your life will not be pushed away.

CHAPTER 15

The Path to Freedom

If freedom came easy to us, then we would not know what it truly means and would take it for granted. The path to freedom is meant to be tough, because that is what makes it so damn great!

FREEDOM IS THE ULTIMATE FEELING. Freedom is what we are all after, isn't it? We all want to freely be our authentic selves, free to do what we love, with financial freedom that allows us to live life and explore the way we do in our dreams.

Your path to personal freedom contains huge mountains of adversity that are deliberately placed in your way. These mountains, though scary, serve a purpose, which is to test your limits, grow your resilience, and teach you lessons that refine your character and prepare you for your destiny.

To back down from these mountains and adversities is choosing to stay stagnant as you opt out of growth. You deny yourself transformation and self-discovery that can only be uncovered by facing such challenges. The mountains are not your enemies; they are your mentors and guides to your destination and lead to your purpose.

Stop playing small because you are scared of adversity. That is you selling yourself short, preventing yourself from uncovering your hidden strengths and untapped potential. Viewing these barriers as a permanent roadblock prevents you from living the life you desire. The struggle that the mountains bring and the effects of your moving those mountains give you real appreciation for the true destination on your path.

Personal freedom is a gift you give yourself, an earned privilege. It's your reward for bravery, persistence, determination, and courage to take adversities head-on and learn the lessons sent to teach and elevate you. You have confronted your doubts and fears and overcome them. Personal freedom shows your unwavering commitment to carving your own path, in order to reach your destiny, even if it previously seemed impossible.

The true suffering lies in choosing the path of least resistance. When you do that, you deprive yourself of feeling the exhilaration and accomplishment of reaching your destination and attaining that sweet taste of personal freedom. You are left with the haunting thoughts of "what if."

Embrace the mountains you encounter on your path to personal freedom. No obstacle can be bigger than your desire for what you seek. When you acknowledge their purpose in preparing you and when you are aware of what they offer, you will remove those mountains much faster, for you know that your destination lies on the other side.

Freedom is the highest level of success. Being successful is so much more than your financial status. True success is having the ability to be your true self with a victor mindset, fulfilling your purpose, loving yourself, and having healthy, fulfilling relationships.

There is a level of success that each of us has in our minds. What separates the ones who achieve that success from those who fail is their willingness to walk through the fires that come their way in the form of hardships, pain, and adversity. Remember, the bigger the fire, the bigger the destiny.

On your path to freedom your mindset will level up as you remove the mountains and break free from the invisible chains and limitations you have put on yourself. Your mindset will transform into a powerful one that will only help you obtain all that you desire. This path empowers you to live authentically, never settling, and always embracing life to the very fullest.

The path of freedom is where you break free and shatter your limiting beliefs that hold you back. This is where you get rid of the thoughts that no longer serve you well, like "I'm not good enough," "I will never achieve it," or "I don't deserve to be happy." Those are simply limitations you have put on yourself that, once removed, will open the door to transformation and self-discovery.

When you have a mindset of freedom, you dream differently. You are wide-open to endless possibilities that you no longer attach fear of failure to. This mindset shift changes how you view adversity. You no longer see them as obstacles but as opportunities to grow and level up. That shift gives you the courage and resilience to take risks on yourself and not give up.

You will learn who you are at your very core, allowing you to be true to your authentic self, which leads you to live authentically, while staying true to your values and beliefs. You free yourself of the invisible chain of living your life to appease others, and instead do what feels right and fulfilling for you.

You will have more meaningful and satisfying relationships, because you will attract others with similar beliefs and mindset. You will have no room in your life for fake people and emotional vampires. You will have deeper connections and a sense of belonging in your relationships, which will only be possible with a mindset free of limiting beliefs.

Life is too short to live in mediocrity. Choose the path of freedom, so you can transform into your true self and unlock your true potential. The benefits of having a mindset of freedom include:

1. **Endless Possibilities:** When you have a mindset of freedom, you dream differently. You are wide-open to endless possibilities that you no longer attach fear of failure to. You view life as an adventure, confident in whatever comes your way.
2. **Authenticity**: You uncover your true, authentic self. This leads you to living authentically and staying true to your values and beliefs. You form deeper and more meaningful connections.
3. **Unbreakable Resilience**: You cannot free your mind without obtaining a deep, permanent resilience. This will give the confidence that, no matter what comes your way, you will come through the other side better than before.

4. **Confidence**: You will be confident in who you are and in all of the decisions you make, never conforming to the status quo. You will stay true to your authentic self.
5. **Health Booster**: A mindset of freedom vastly improves your emotional and mental well-being. When you rid yourself of negative thoughts, you remove a lot of stress and anxiety. You help your immune system to stay strong, and overall, you feel better from the inside out.
6. **Super Attractor**: A mindset of freedom makes you a super attractor! We attract what we embody, and we become magnets based on the energy we put out.
7. **Stay in Your Power**: The mindset of freedom is empowering. You take charge of your own destiny, and you control the reins on your path to success.
8. **Life of Fulfillment**: A mindset of freedom is a life of purpose and fulfillment. You can reflect and know that you lived authentically to your full potential, making the very most of your time here on Earth.

A mindset of freedom is the most powerful tool for living the most fulfilling, rewarding life one can live. It is the only way to live authentically and free, fulfilling your purpose and doing what you love.

Get Real Uncomfortable

The path to freedom requires you to be uncomfortable. Remember, we grow in discomfort! People do not like to be uncomfortable. In fact, as humans we go out of our way to be comfortable, super-comfortable. We want everything at the drop of a hat, delivered to us, waited on, not too cold, not too hot, extra-soft blankets, super-soft bed, pain medicine for pain, and anti-anxiety meds for anxiety. Are you picking up what I am putting down?

The cold, hard truth is that growth is not possible in comfort, and comfort does not exist in growth. It is within the discomfort, where we are stretched and molded, pushed outside of our familiar boundaries, that we are able to become our true selves. And, if you choose to stay comfortable, then you can never tap into your true potential.

Never settle in the confines of comfort, getting stuck where you feel safe. You lose your motivation to do more and be more. The arms of comfort become an anchor to your growth as you become scared to step out of it and explore anything that is different. It is easy to become complacent in our routines and choices. We are creatures of habit, and we like what is familiar to us. It makes us feel safe.

As you steer clear of discomfort, you also steer clear of change, denying yourself the opportunity to grow and evolve. Discomfort exercises and tests our resilience, enhances our adaptability, and promotes self-discovery. Left unexercised, we become weak and a prisoner to ourselves.

In contrast, it is in the discomfort that we find the ingredients for transformation. It is there that our minds can become free of limiting beliefs, fears, and insecurities, giving us a new free mindset, new perspectives, and new strengths that we didn't even know we had. As we face challenges and overcome them, we are shaped and molded into exactly what we need to embody in order to fulfill our purpose.

Every obstacle, every challenge, and every adversity is an opportunity to uncover yourself and your hidden potential.

The discomfort is where you find out what you are really made of.

The true detriment is staying stuck in the grip of comfort and eventually being tortured by the thoughts of what could have been, if you hadn't stayed confined to comfort. It is a life lived without fulfillment and joy.

In the end, discomfort is your key to growth and transformation. Comfort is your anchor to mediocrity and your sentence to an unfulfilling life. So, embrace the discomfort, the challenges, and the uncertainty as your teachers that will transform you into your authentic self. Every time you are hesitant about breaking out of your comfort zone, I want you to remember what the consequences are of staying there. Remind yourself that getting uncomfortable is the ingredient to growth.

We go out of our way to make living life as comfortable as possible, so if we have the choice to *pull out of anything that is making us uncomfortable,* we will do so! However, if you cannot endure the discomfort on the path to freedom, then you will never obtain it. This is where *free will* comes in!

What is the number-one reason you or anyone quit something they were once going after? Discomfort, my friends. Discomfort comes in many forms, like:
- ✓ Rejection
- ✓ Fear
- ✓ Intimidation
- ✓ Self-defeat
- ✓ Failure
- ✓ Insecurities

You do not have to go through the discomfort of healing. Anytime you can exit or eject out of discomfort, that's the choice you will make. The Universe brings seasons to our lives that bring such discomfort where we do not have an eject button, and we cannot exit. We are forced to be uncomfortable, because we grow in discomfort.

The caveat is you can choose to stay in that difficult storm of a season, numbing yourself to not feel the discomfort. *You cannot be forced to grow; it is up to you!* The Universe definitely will push you to rock-bottom, trying to get you to open your eyes, snap out of the victim mentality, and get promoted to the next level.

Where do you feel uncomfortable? Ask yourself these questions:
- ❖ Do new ideas make you uncomfortable that seem impossible?
- ❖ Does the growth and success of others make you uncomfortable?
- ❖ Does facing your unhealed wounds to heal and shattering limiting beliefs make you uncomfortable?
- ❖ Are you uncomfortable being yourself around people?
- ❖ Does the thought of what others will think or say about you, if you live your life the way you want to, make you uncomfortable?
- ❖ Does it make you uncomfortable to think you might continue to live your life on autopilot, unhappy and unfulfilled?

Just three short years ago, I would have answered *yes* to all six of those questions. I was exactly where you are right now. If you are wondering how long it took me to go through the process of shattering limiting beliefs, healing, growing, evolving, and transforming, it took four solid, straight years, plus the two years of learning about mindset shifts, when I was sick with Lyme. So, almost six years! Sounds like a lot, but looking back, it wasn't. It was, however, completely worth it!

Do you want to be comfortable in the discomfort of never knowing what you are capable of? Or do you want to get uncomfortable, so you can be comfortably all that you were meant to be?

It is not going to happen overnight. A caterpillar does not transform into a beautiful butterfly overnight, either. It takes a lot of work internally to stay on the path to freedom. The road to healing and overcoming gets a little bumpy sometimes, but the payoff and reward are more than worth it.

My favorite aphorism, something my kids probably know by heart: "Time goes by no matter what. You can either look back and be really happy, or you can look back and wish you would have." That's it. Those are your two choices.

My rewards for shattering my limiting beliefs, healing, forgiving, and unf*cking my mind are not temporary or short lived. My rewards:
- ❖ I no longer live my life trying to fill voids.
- ❖ I no longer live my life looking in the rearview mirror. Only straight ahead.
- ❖ I love myself, accept who I am, and approve of myself. I no longer need anyone's approval.
- ❖ I face fear head-on, while allowing myself to feel the discomfort, so I can understand why and then overcome it.
- ❖ I am fulfilling my purpose.

The purpose of choosing the path of freedom in our mindset is to break free from limiting beliefs, live authentically, and embrace all of possibilities that life has to offer. It empowers us to take control of our lives, pursue our dreams, stop settling, create a sense of fulfillment that only comes from living a life true to our authentic selves. While the journey toward a mindset of freedom may not be easy, the rewards it offers are well worth any discomfort you encounter.

So, what do you have to lose? Choose the path of freedom, and embark on this journey that leads you to the life you want to live and that is full of purpose.

There is a profound truth about life that is both freeing and empowering: the power we all have to choose the paths we take in our lives. We often give that power away to everyone else to choose our fate, and we don't even realize sometimes that we actually have a choice.

You do not have to lie down and accept the so-called fate that comes your way through adversities, diagnosis, and challenges. You get to choose what you accept and what action you take to overcome it. For the longest time, I accepted every little thing and thought that came into my life, assuming it was just my luck. But the moment when I realized that I had the power to choose and change my trajectory in life was huge!

The path to your personal growth lies in your very own hands. This truth is the key to unlocking your true potential. Your life is your personal book, and you are the author of it. You might not be able to go back and rewrite your past, but there are blank pages waiting to be filled by the choices you make. You can now write the rest of your story exactly the way you dream it. Every decision and choice you make from here on out determines what story you write.

In understanding this power, you then acknowledge that, regardless of your external circumstances or past experiences, your present and future are determined by the choices and decisions you make now, and those hold the key to your future. So, shed the victim mindset, break the invisible chains holding you back, shatter the limiting beliefs that have worn out their welcome, and step into your power without apologizing for it.

Knowing that you have the power to choose and grow in life is a profound awakening. It gives you a sense of responsibility that pushes you to make decisions with intention and purpose. You must step into the role of being the creator of your own reality and no one else.

With every choice and decision, you are shaping your destiny. So, make choices and decisions from this moment forward that are aligned with your values and beliefs and that promote the growth you seek. Choosing to grow is intentional and deliberate, so always be intentional and deliberate with every decision you make, based on the kind of life you want to live.

In the end, the importance of recognizing that you have the power to choose and grow in life is solely in your hands, and it is up to you to exercise that right. Embrace this power that resides in you, and choose to take the path to freedom. Realize that you will write your own story from now on, never giving anyone the pen, and live by your own damn rules.

*****

Takeaway: *Take a step, take a leap of faith, but take a chance on yourself.*

CHAPTER 16

Say Yes to You!

Be more afraid of not being authentically who you truly are than of showing your true self! You must first choose yourself and then the Universe follows, opening the door for everything else to say yes to you.

HOW DO YOU FEEL, having almost read this entire book? It is a lot to soak in, so give yourself the space to do so. I recommend reading this book again, after you have self-reflected and given your brain time to absorb all of these new concepts, ideas, and realizations.

Throughout life, there are an insurmountable number of choices that unfold before us, but there is one decision that serves as a transformative turning point in our lives. The decision of saying yes to yourself. This is a decision that holds the power to reshape the course of your existence, to unlock the doors to your true self, and to put you on the path of self-discovery that leads you to your destination.

Saying yes to yourself is you shouting out to the Universe that you believe in yourself and that you are worth it. You don't need that validation from one damn person except yourself. It is the moment you choose to go after your dreams, desires, and purpose, above all else. You are no longer putting yourself and dreams on the back burner. It is you recognizing that your happiness, choice of fulfillment, and your purpose are of upmost importance.

Making this decision is not easy, and it takes a deep desire to live an authentic life filled with fulfillment. You are announcing that you are deserving of a life that aligns with your true self, free from the expectations and judgments of others. This is the first courageous step toward embracing your uniqueness and authentic self.

To say yes to yourself is to step on the path of freedom and to your destiny. It is a step of self-empowerment, a commitment to growth and transformation, and to no longer hide your talents. You are making a promise to yourself to invest in yourself and in what you believe in, regardless of outside opinions.

You are stepping into your independence and power when you choose yourself. You are no longer afraid to confront challenges and adversities, but rather aware of the reward in confronting them and what it offers. You know that life's challenges are merely a means to your personal freedom.

There is a powerful effect when you say yes to yourself that is more than just making that statement. There is a domino effect that touches every single part of your life that leaves nothing the same as before. It gives you the power to make the changes in your life that are necessary for your new journey. You are able to set boundaries, make choices that align with your values and desires, and live intentionally with purpose. You no longer feel like you are living your life like a hamster on a hamster wheel.

It is a life-changing decision of saying yes to yourself, the ultimate act of self-love, self-acceptance, and self-worth. It affirms that your existence here on Earth is your story to tell and you are the sole author of it. Your life ahead is a blank canvas, and you hold the pen. Your actions moving forward will not be influenced by anyone or anything other than your desires and dreams.

Are you ready to say yes to yourself? If not, what is holding you back? Maybe you feel that you are too different. Or maybe there is someone else already doing exactly what you want to do, and they are successful at it, so there is no point in you trying?

If that is the case, you could be dealing with imposter syndrome, which is exactly how it sounds. This is very common and can come up from time to time, no matter how successful you might be.

What exactly does imposter syndrome feel like? It creates this nagging feeling of self-doubt, making you feel inadequate. It is extremely common and entirely normal, when you step out of your comfort zone and into unchartered territory that you are seeking. Even the most successful and accomplished people feel imposter syndrome from time to time and struggle with it.

However, imposter syndrome is simply a fear and insecurity we create in our mind because of the expectations we put on ourselves and ones from the outside world. Anytime we are stepping into a new career or season of our life, it can create uncertainty of the outcome we seek. So, as you navigate uncharted territory, if imposter syndrome hits, remember it is perfectly normal. These reminders will help you get past imposter syndrome.

1. **Comfort Zone**: You moved out of your comfort zone, so it is normal to feel uneasy, questioning where you are. Remember, you grow in the discomfort.
2. **Expectations**: Do not set high expectations for yourself. Also, the expectation of needing to know what the outcome will be is not possible. Never expect yourself to be at the level of those who have been doing it for much longer. Do not compare yourself to anyone.
3. **Fears and Insecurities**: Insecurities and fears are made-up feelings of imposter syndrome. They are not real, so do not give in.
4. **Perfectionism**: Remember that perfectionism is not achievable. You are perfectly imperfect.
5. **Validation**: You do not need validation of the new path and journey you are on. You only need to validate your own damn self.

Imposter syndrome is a normal response when stepping out of your comfort zone. It feels incredibly liberating and means you're taking risks, pursuing growth, and pushing yourself. View it as a sign that you're stepping outside of your boundaries and striving for more in your life.

Rather than seeing imposter syndrome as an obstacle, view it as a teacher on your journey. It's a reminder that you're growing and transforming on this path of self-discovery. These feelings don't define you. Remember that even successful people face imposter syndrome at some point and it can rear its ugly head from time to time.

Imposter syndrome creates thoughts like:

> - I am not good enough.
> - Someone else is already doing it and better.
> - No one will listen to me, like me, or want to work with me.
> - I have nothing else to give in that area, because other people have said/done it already.
> - I don't think I have enough experience.

If any of those thoughts weigh you down and keep you from letting your light shine, then please stop! I have struggled with imposter syndrome, and guess what? I still do sometimes. But I quickly remind myself that no one else has my voice.

Repeat after me: "*No one else has my voice!*"

That's right. Say it as much as you need to, as a reminder that you are unique, and it is *your* uniqueness that makes you different. Let that sink in! You need to let your uniqueness shine. The world needs your light, my friend.

When I first struggled with this syndrome, I was just stepping into where I am now and was around a bunch of super-successful, beautiful, well-known women who were already doing everything I wanted to do. And to top it off, they were doing a damn good job. I am pretty sure you could hear me swallow when I stepped into the room with these women. I wanted to crawl underneath the table and hide. Seriously.

Here are the exact thoughts that went through my head at that moment: "They're going to know I am new, and I don't have all their years of experience. Who is going to read my book? Who am I to write the book? My podcast will never be as big as theirs. I will never have a huge following like them. They already know the ins and outs, and there is no way I can say anything better than they do."

We all have a voice. You have a voice, and it needs to be heard!

What makes me so special and different is my uniqueness. What makes you so special and different is your uniqueness. There are many nutritionists, podcasters, authors, and speakers out there, but none of our voices are the same. The way we write, the way we think, the way we talk are all different. The reason why is that none of us have the same life experiences and interpretations. There are tons of nutritionists who once dealt with major gut issues and healed their gut. However, their experience and interpretation of it will not be the same as mine, and they will not teach it the same way!

I said *no* to myself for way too long, and *no* to what makes me unique. I am so very grateful that I embraced all that makes me unique and for saying *yes* to myself. It is time for you to do the same! Stop worrying about what others think. You need to worry about what you think of yourself. Get in alignment with what God thinks of you, and everything else will fall into place. Doing so will activate your powers and tell the universe that you are ready. You are ready to do what it is that you were put on Earth to do.

Never change one damn thing that makes you unique and stand out, because no one else has what you have. There is not one other person like me or you. We are all uniquely different and for a reason. Stop hiding. Be who you are. Do what you feel called to do.

The Power of Alone Time

You can hear the whispers in the silence.

Making time to be alone with yourself is imperative to your growth and evolution. Do you ever have true alone time by yourself? No kids, friends, family, or partner. Just you. As you have reached the end of this book, I want to teach you one last thing. It will be so helpful in your healing journey.

Life is full of demands, obligations, relationships, deadlines, and responsibilities. We all have them, and we are all busy with way too much on our plates. However, we all make time for the things we want to do. It is easy to give the excuse that we don't have time on our schedule, but that is bullshit. You can always make time for yourself and your well-being. If you don't, then all of the demands and obligations in your life are going to suffocate you. So, how do you fix that?

Alone time. Make room in your schedule for alone time. This sacred time for yourself is imperative for your growth, health, and emotional well-being. This is what allows you to check-in with yourself, self-reflect, and discover. It allows you to hit pause in your frantic schedule. It is the moment when the world's demands take a backseat to your self-care. You are able to give yourself space to be with your own thoughts, desires, and emotions.

The power of alone time offers:
1. **Self-Reflection**: Alone time allows you to reflect on your thoughts and emotions. You can reflect on your

experiences and fears to help you gain a deeper understanding of yourself and where you are.
2. **Recalibrate**: Without alone time, it is easy to fall into the routine of a schedule and demands, which can lead to stagnation. Alone time allows you pull yourself out of the weeds and remember what your goals are, so you can reset yourself.
3. **Ignite Creativity**: Alone time is the igniter of creativity. It is in the quiet moments, when we are by ourselves, that our mind can let go of our to-do list and venture off into exploration. This was huge for me, personally, in writing this book.
4. **Revive**: In the quiet time, we can process our feelings, release any pent-up emotions, and return to our inner peace. This is your opportunity for healing and emotional attunement.
5. **Clarity and Focus**: Alone time provides the mental space to untangle the variables thrown our way that can blur our vision to what we truly seek. It allows you to see your obstacles clearly without external influence and make decisions without distractions.
6. **Nurture Growth**: The power of alone time is imperative for personal growth. This is when you can recognize limitations you have set or fears blocking your way. This allows you to confront them and remove them.
7. **Enhance Relationships**: Having alone time, in a healthy way, can surprisingly enhance your relationships. It allows you to take a step back and evaluate your relationships and where they may be

lacking. We get so comfortable in relationships that we take them for granted. Alone time allows you and your partner to stay in touch with your own needs and desires, allowing you to communicate more effectively and have more fulfilling connections.

8. **Reconnecting**: The power of alone time gives room to reconnect with yourself and who you are. It is easy to lose our sense of self in the demands of our lives. When you lose the ability to think for yourself, you can lose your identity. Alone time allows you to reconnect with yourself, nature, and your purpose.

Alone time is the only way you can truly be with yourself. Your only companion is yourself. This is a special time of self-discovery, a time to renew your strength, to reconnect with yourself, and an opportunity for soul searching.

Not nearly enough people give themselves true alone time. Some even frown upon it or make fun of it, and some are scared to be alone with themselves. I want to make something very clear: being alone is not the same thing as being lonely. So, do not confuse the two.

Being alone with yourself allows you to breathe, self-reflect, and feel all that you feel without interruption. It was in the alone time that I could work on my healing during Lyme and the divorce. It was in the alone time where I found myself, my power, my worth, and my boundaries.

Do not feel guilty for asking for alone time. Some of you are single, while some have a partner, kids, families, you name it. I promise, you can make time for alone time. If anyone makes you feel guilty or weird for needing it, well, they are a weed, and you know what to do with them. The right people who truly love you will want to give you this space and will probably even be happy you asked for it! Get rid of the idea that you need to be everything to everyone all the time. That is impossible, and you are going to wear yourself out. It seems like we are running a race, trying to catch our breath. But how can you catch your breath if you never stop?

We all get so consumed with being busy and having schedules that our lives turn into chaos 24/7. You end up with a calendar full of events, activities, sports, meetings, and social gatherings, because you do not want to let anyone down. You know what? You are letting yourself down.

How can you be 100% for yourself and what matters the most (kids and partner), if you are giving it away everywhere else? Stop trying to balance it all and appease everyone. You are the one suffering. And when you suffer, it just trickles down into your kids, partner, and career. You have to be willing to give up mediocrity in order to gain prosperity. Giving yourself alone time is creating a boundary for yourself. Remember that boundaries keep the weeds out and allow us to bloom.

There is no wrong way to have alone time. Sometimes, it is only an hour or so, and other times, it is for six hours or a whole day. Take what you can get. Just make sure you get it. If you put it in your mind that it needs to be over a certain amount of time, then you will end up depriving yourself of precious time. It all counts and adds up. We make time in our schedules for everyone and everything without fail, so we can do the same for ourselves, can't we?

To clear up any confusion, here is what alone time is *not*:

- ✓ Happy hour with a friend(s)
- ✓ Making phone call after phone call, if you can't see your friends.
- ✓ Obsessively scrolling social media for a distraction
- ✓ Working
- ✓ Chores

Every single one of those is a distraction! The purpose of alone time with yourself is to not be distracted, because you are 24/7! This is your time to recenter yourself, get in touch with your feelings, reflect, breathe, heal, and relax. This is one of the best forms of self-care.

Yes, the spa, massages, yoga, and Pilates are great, but nothing is going to do more for you than being alone with yourself. This is where you recharge your battery, so you do not get drained. It is really hard to give and do with a dead battery or on an empty tank.

I look forward to my alone time. I no longer feel guilty about it. I am honest about it. I am a better me, mother, and wife, when I get time to reflect. It is really hard, almost impossible, to self-reflect, if you are not by yourself. I can tell when I am overdue for it, because I begin to feel overwhelmed and get a little cranky. My husband now knows exactly what I need. Sometimes, we have to pull ourselves out of the cycle of life, so we can see it from the outside looking in!

Alone time by yourself allows you to breathe without the pressure, demands, and needs of others. Especially if you are a parent! A fire goes out, if it is deprived of oxygen. It has to breathe. Guess what? It is the exact same for you! Your fire will go out, if you do not get a chance to breathe. Hell, maybe your fire isn't even lit or the flame is dim. If that is the case, then the only way to ignite your fire is to do the inner work, shatter your limiting beliefs, and heal your wounds and insecurities. Through that, you will find exactly what lights your fire!

Reflection

Reflection is a powerful tool. It allows us to explore our thoughts, emotions, and experiences. To peel back the layers and discover who we truly are. It also is how we can check in with ourselves and evaluate decisions, actions, intentions, and our direction. As I said previously, one of the reasons alone time is so powerful is because it allows for self-reflection.

Life is a roller-coaster ride, full of ups and downs, twists and turns. We get so caught up in the craziness of our lives, we forget to stop and smell the roses. We lose sight of what really matters. We get sucked into the obligations and demands of our calendar, which always seems to be full.

Alone time offers reflection. Making space to self-reflect is how you gain clarity and perspective on where you are in life, your goals and purpose. This is where you can find courage to make the necessary changes to create the life you want to live.

Do not confuse reflection with a time to dwell on the past or get stuck in regret. That is not at all what reflection is. It's about learning from your experiences, being aware of your behavior and feelings, seeing your improvements, and embracing your growth. It is the only way you can see yourself and your life from the "outside looking in."

So how can you incorporate reflection into your life? By making it a priority and not a "when you get time" task, which never gets done. Whether it's through journaling, meditation, or simply taking a walk-in nature, find what works for you.

The only requirement is that you are alone, and your phone is on silent or in another room.

Give yourself permission to disconnect from the outside world and reconnect with yourself. Never feel guilty for giving yourself this time or allow others to make you feel guilty for doing so. Remind yourself and others that having alone time to reflect makes you a better you. Reflection helps you to uncover your passions, values, and purpose. You are able to gain a deeper understanding of yourself and what truly brings you joy and fulfillment.

Reflection is not just a one-time activity that solves your problems. It is an ongoing practice. It is a tool to use throughout your life to ignite self-discovery and personal growth. Self-reflection is a powerful tool for staying true to your authentic self and in alignment with your beliefs, desires, and purpose. It is having the ability to look inward and examine where you are in that present moment and where you are headed.

Here are several benefits of self-reflection what it offers for personal growth:

1. **Self-Awareness:** Self-reflection keeps you in tune with your thoughts, feelings, and behaviors. You are able to identify patterns, and it enables you to notice the areas you may want to change or improve. You are able to clarify your beliefs and core values.
2. **Internal Check-In:** Self-reflection gives you the ability to check in with your emotions, goals, and any problems that might be going on. You are able to identify obstacles, gauge progress, develop strategies, and identify any emotional triggers.

3. **Strengthen Relationships:** You are able to reflect on your interactions and communications with others. You can more clearly see the impact you have on others and where improvements can be made. You are able to develop better communication and listening skills. This helps strengthen and deepen your connections, making them more meaningful.
4. **Improved Empathy:** When we are able to take a step back and reflect, not only on our lives, but on those around us, we are able to empathize with what others are going through. Sometimes, we are so close to what is going on, we are not able to truly see the effect a situation is having on those we love.
5. **Fosters a Growth Mindset:** Self-reflection fosters a growth mindset. As you reflect on your past experiences and how you handled them, you are able to recognize where you can improve and do things differently. This is also what allows you to see how much you have grown, by comparing how you handled past challenges and failures. This perspective builds your resilience and a more optimistic outlook on growth.
6. **Accountability:** Self-reflection allows you to more clearly see areas in your life where you need to be more accountable and responsible for your actions and decisions. In doing so, you can make necessary changes and avoid repeating past mistakes. This sense of accountability ensures continued personal growth and not falling into a victim mindset.

Self-reflection is imperative for personal growth. When you regularly have alone time, you are able to engage in self-reflection. This helps you to stay in a growth mindset, strengthen and deepen connections, and stay in tune with yourself. It motivates you to overcome challenges, pursue your goals, and lead a more fulfilling life. Self-reflection enables self-discovery, which leads to increased self-awareness, more empathy, and adaptability, and ensures a mindset of growth.

Choose You

You have made it to the end of this book. Do you feel like you are in a rut, not able to reach your full potential? If so, it's time to break free from this mindset and unlock the power within you. It all starts with a simple shift in perspective. A mindset shift that changes everything. It's about embracing a positive and growth-oriented mindset.

Instead of looking at challenges as obstacles, see them as opportunities for personal growth. Every setback is a chance to learn and improve. By cultivating a growth mindset, you become more resilient, adaptable, and confident. You'll start seeing setbacks as stepping stones to success.

Remember, your thoughts create your reality. When you believe in yourself and your abilities, you have the power to achieve greatness. No longer held back by limiting beliefs, you'll start taking risks, stepping out of your comfort zone, and unleashing your full potential. So, how do you shift your mindset? It's about being mindful of your thoughts and actively replacing negative self-talk with positive affirmations.

The older I got, the more I felt I was never going to find my purpose. Age does not matter. Don't put requirements and limitations on yourself, because the moment you do, you stop trying. It didn't matter what I was thinking on some made up timeline I created for my dreams. All that mattered was I had said yes to me and took action.

The choice followed by action was all the Universe was waiting for. I just didn't know it. God's plan for us is much bigger than ours. I am still in disbelief that it all happened in one year, and all I did was choose myself for the first time ever.

God had everything lined up as if it was right there and in place. Remember, within one week, I came across my mentor, who is now so much more than that. She is also a dear friend and a true angel in my life. She believed in me when I really had nothing to show for it. I just believed in myself. You will attract what you embody. Let that sink in.

The stars aligned beautifully for me in that pivotal moment that changed the course of my life forever. It was the moment when I finally believed in myself. The moment when I had the courage to say "yes" to myself. For way too long, I'd lived my life and made decisions based on others' expectations. I'd gone out of my way to fit into their molds and ideas of how I should be and what I should do. I had too long ignored the whispers of my inner voice, the voice that knew my authentic self, passions, and purpose. I'd allowed the influence from others to drown out my own dreams.

Thank goodness I finally had the realization and chose to invest in myself, say yes to myself, and finally believe in all that I was and am. I was nervous and scared of the unknown, of the new beginnings. This time, though, I wasn't nervous or scared out of fear; it was out of excitement about what was to come and of knowing that I had opened doors to my dreams and purpose. It was as if the Universe had just been waiting for me to choose myself.

The moment I said "yes," a strong feeling of empowerment filled me, telling me that I was on the right path. It was like nothing I had ever felt before. My energy felt renewed, I felt stronger, and I had a strong gut feeling that I was closer than ever to living the life I had always dreamed of. My eyes flooded with tears as I reflected on every single heartache, adversity, and pain I had chosen to overcome, which had made me who I was in that very moment. I was no longer angry at the strength I'd once wished would go away, but rather more grateful for it than ever before. I embraced and understood why I'd had to go through such difficult times and how they'd groomed and molded me into all that I was.

I felt the release of every invisible chain that had once held me back and the shattering of limiting beliefs that had once held me prisoner in my own mind. The result of overcoming what could have been my detriment was that it was the key to unlocking the doors to my purpose here on Earth.

I felt pure freedom in that moment. Free from the expectations of others, the pressure of society, limiting beliefs, and fears. I felt free from the inside out. Free to be my true authentic self without a care about what anyone else thought of me. I was completely and wholly happy, which I had never felt before. I knew that, no matter what came my way, nothing or no one could take my happiness, confidence, or self-worth.

About all of those moments from my past, when I had wondered why something was happening to me and couldn't understand what possible good could ever come of it, I no longer was confused. It was very clear why I'd had to walk through every one of those storms. I was grateful for all of them and the lessons they'd brought me.

Every locked door came unlocked as I continued saying "yes" to myself. The connections I began and continue to make are deeper and richer than I ever could have had without going on this journey of the path to freedom. I now embrace the challenges that come my way as opportunities for growth. I no longer question setbacks. Rather, I know the Universe is showing me something or protecting me from what I cannot see.

Today, my heart is overflowing with gratitude. I am living the life I was meant to live, the one I once dreamt of. I am fulfilling my purpose, and I am confident in my ability to handle all that comes my way. My eyes are wide-open to how the Universe works, why we are presented with "lessons", and the reward for learning them.

The power of your mind is your determining factor to what level of success you will reach in every single aspect of your life. It is mind-blowing, how much we cannot see when we are blinded by fears, limiting beliefs, pain, and insecurities. I can easily see when someone is being held back by their mindset, but I never could have noticed that before I healed my own. No one should live as a prisoner in their own mind, held back by invisible chains.

Tell me, what are you waiting for? What excuse are you giving yourself? No one can make it happen for you other than your own damn self. Your purpose awaits, and it is a journey worth taking, but only you can make that decision.

Just don't blame anyone else but yourself, if you are not living the life you desire. Start saying "yes." The rewards are more than worth it, and so are you. My rewards have come in so many forms, and they will keep coming, because I will never stop saying "yes" to myself.

I finally have unconditional love from a partner. I am madly in love with my husband, and my kids have an amazing bonus dad. I feel the true happiness and fulfillment I always wanted. I look forward to all that life has in store for me, and I am not scared. I want the same for you. You deserve the same.

I share all my accomplishments with you as I have shared my struggles and adversities. I have poured my heart and soul into every word you are holding, to show others they can do the same and that anything is possible, when you have a victory mentality. I have given all of me in this book. Now, you have to do the rest. You must choose, so choose *you*! Say yes to you, and say out loud, "I deserve it!"

My stories of overcoming on my journey to get to where I am today are proof of all that is possible, when you shatter limiting beliefs, shift your mindset, and say yes to yourself. I got sick and tired of being told what I was capable of and what I should do. I allowed others to put limits on me. The day I took the pen back, I began rewriting my own story. It's time to rewrite your story. You have the power to create the life you've always dreamed of. Believe in yourself. Embrace the power of mindset.

You are not meant to live your life, barely shining your light. You are meant to shine your light bright, my friend! The world needs you, and only light can drown out the darkness.

Thank you for taking your time to read this book. Shine that light, baby!

With much love, gratitude, and appreciation,

Janna

ACKNOWLEDGMENTS

I AM DEEPLY GRATEFUL to the many individuals who have played a significant role in the creation of this book. Your support, encouragement, and expertise have been invaluable throughout this journey.

I want to thank my husband, my three precious kids, and my family for their unwavering support and understanding during the long hours I spent writing. Your love and encouragement sustained me.

I am deeply grateful to my husband, Brent, for his undying patience, understanding, and love. You have given me the best gift a person could want from their partner: unconditional love. You understand me like no other, and you are my best friend. I love you with all of me for eternity.

To my dear friends, your belief in me and your encouragement, whether through a listening ear or a kind word, helped me persevere when doubt crept in. Jennifer, your constant prayers and support are unwavering.

I am indebted to Amberly Lago for her invaluable guidance, wisdom, friendship, and mentorship. Her expertise and belief in me and my work were instrumental in shaping this book. Amberly, you are such an inspiration and light to me and so many others. I love you and appreciate you so very much.

I want to extend my gratitude to Samantha Joy, my publisher, for her keen insights and patience throughout the writing process. Her belief in me and her wisdom brought my journey to life with this book. Thank you, Samantha, for believing in me and bringing out this book that was in me, that I wasn't even aware of. You are an inspiration to me.

I'd like to acknowledge the publishing team at Landon Hail Press for their professionalism and support in bringing this book to life. I enjoy working with all of you and look forward to more.

Lastly, I express my gratitude to the readers who will soon embark on this literary journey. Your interest in my work means the world to me.

Writing this book has been a labor of love, and I am profoundly thankful to each of you for being a part of it. Your contributions, no matter how big or small, have left an indelible mark on this work.

Thank you for believing in me and this book.

Janna Johnson

ABOUT THE AUTHOR

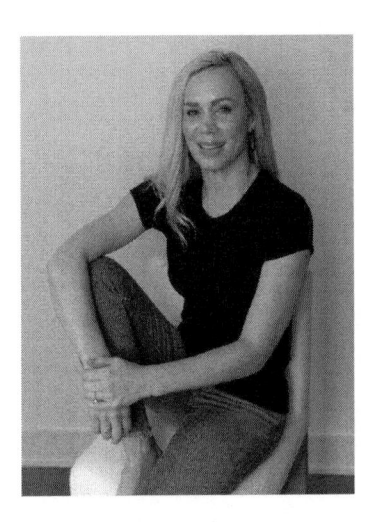

JANNA JOHNSON IS A renowned mindset coach, accomplished nutritionist, and a beacon of inspiration in the world of personal development. Her journey is nothing short of remarkable; having overcome the challenges of Lyme disease, she not only healed herself 100% but also discovered the incredible power of the human mind. Today, Janna Johnson is on a mission to share her wisdom and experiences to help others transform their lives.

In a story of resilience and determination, Janna conquered Lyme disease, defying the odds and regaining her health against all expectations. Her personal battle with this debilitating illness has given her unique insights into the mind-body connection and the importance of a positive mindset in the healing process.

With a deep understanding that mindset is the cornerstone of all success in life, Janna has dedicated herself to coaching individuals to unlock their full potential. Her expertise as a nutritionist complements her work, which emphasizes a holistic approach to well-being, where a healthy body and a strong mind go hand in hand.

Janna's first book, *Unf*ck Your Mind,* is a powerful guide designed to help readers shatter limiting beliefs that may be holding them back. Drawing from her personal triumphs and professional expertise, it provides actionable strategies to empower individuals to overcome obstacles, achieve their goals, and lead fulfilling lives.

Janna's inspiring journey, coupled with her dedication to personal development and transformation, makes her a sought-after speaker, coach, and author in the field of mindset and wellness. Her mission is to empower others to embrace the limitless potential of their minds and bodies and to lead lives filled with purpose, vitality, and success.

If you are interested in learning more about Janna Johnson's courses and coaching, how to tune into her podcast, *Revive with Janna*, or if you are looking for a keynote speaker for your next event, please visit:

www.revivebyjanna.com

Or follow her on Instagram:
@ReviveByJanna

Made in the USA
Middletown, DE
29 January 2024